THE
SLEEP
SOLUTION

'Sleep is a source of prana—healing, relaxing, rejuvenating—providing subtle energy to the body and mind. Along with the waking, the dreaming and the meditative, it is one of the four states of consciousness. Understanding sleep can unlock many secrets of our consciousness'—Gurudev Sri Sri Ravi Shankar, spiritual leader and founder, the Art of Living Foundation

'We take sleep for granted, until, over the years, you acquire a lifestyle when we spend minimal time sleeping. It doesn't come when you want it to come or comes leaving others around you sleepless! I have always concerned myself with alternate ways of healing and, through this, I have been drawn to breathing. Breathing—which is most essential to all humans and the most natural of all biological functions—begins to evade us in almost the same way as sleep. Thus, how we breathe when we're asleep becomes a vital concern and an important area of study. I had begun to snore and, like most men, ignored it for years until it became unbearable for my wife, Meera. She soon discovered the cause of this disorder. Erratic breathing and stopping of the breath while sleeping pose huge dangers. This is when I approached Dr Manvir Bhatia and have not looked back since. I don't mind sleeping with a breathing apparatus and find a positive change in my overall metabolism—sort of an equivalent to an all-night pranayama session. More than that, my wife now sleeps really well'—Muzaffar Ali, film-maker, poet, artist

'An important, thought-provoking and, ultimately, necessary book on the importance of sleep for our mental, emotional and physical well-being. In *The Sleep Solution*, Dr Manvir Bhatia explains why we are so tired all the time and what we can do to change it. As we sleepwalk into a global sleep crisis, this book will prove an invaluable resource for anyone who wants to get a good night's rest'—Dr Naresh Trehan, chairman, managing director and chief cardiac surgeon, Medanta – The Medicity

'Manvir Bhatia's *The Sleep Solution* offers a fascinating insight into a world over which we often lose so much sleep. The ultimate yardstick of success is not money or fame, but a good night's rest and Bhatia delves into this domain with tremendous academic panache, and years of research and practical experience. Don't go to bed without reading this. Because if you do, you won't ever know what happens when your eyes are shut. Wonderfully written in a manner that is bereft of jargon, and is, instead, extremely simple and measured'—Suhel Seth, managing partner, Counselage India

'We have always given the utmost importance to our waking hours—our activities, work, hobbies, aspirations, career, etc. crowd that time. Yet, little do we realize that sleep forms nearly one-third of our lives and it is the most important activity that we all do for our survival. This excellent book by Dr Manvir Bhatia not only reminds us about the importance of sleep, but provides solutions for a good night's rest. It is perhaps one of the most important reads for all of us to be healthy and happy, because our bodies require a good night's rest to perform well. Poor sleep results in numerous illnesses, from something as simple as irritability and poor concentration to high blood pressure, obesity, heart disease and even death. Thus, we owe it to ourselves and our bodies to enjoy a good night's rest through the solutions in Dr Bhatia's book. It would help, prevent and treat many serious illnesses, and help us stay fit'—Dr Ashok Seth, Padma Bhushan and Padma Shri awardee; chairman, Fortis Escorts Heart Institute

'It is a delight to read a doctor's professional take on sleep. And she is not just any doctor, but one who, I suspect, lost some sleep on my account! Dr Manvir Bhatia has produced a book that's a testimony to her dedication to a subject that occupies (or at least it should) one-third of our lives. Sleep deprivation is a form of torture used in the Gulag or at Guantanamo Bay. But we're increasingly inflicting it upon ourselves through the kind of stressful social structures we opt to live in, and the ever-increasing threat from the "blue-light radiance" off the multiple devices, which have become extensions of our lives. Even more unnoticed is the dominance and prevalence of light pollution in our lives. We are, today, co-creating physical disharmony and mental imbalance on a scale that's not quite measured. Understanding sleep is among the many things Dr Bhatia has mastered. Once you absorb the salient points of her book, you will learn when and why you must be alerted to your own sleep pattern. And you get to know what to do about it and how to ensure that your errors don't alter the pattern of the "rest that restores". Grab this book, absorb it and then sleep deep!'—Dilip Cherian, co-founder and consulting partner, Perfect Relations

THE
SLEEP
SOLUTION

SECRETS FOR A
GOOD NIGHT'S SLEEP

DR MANVIR BHATIA

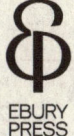

EBURY
PRESS
An imprint of Penguin Random House

EBURY PRESS

USA | Canada | UK | Ireland | Australia
New Zealand | India | South Africa | China | Singapore

Ebury Press is part of the Penguin Random House group of companies
whose addresses can be found at global.penguinrandomhouse.com

Published by Penguin Random House India Pvt. Ltd
4th Floor, Capital Tower 1, MG Road,
Gurugram 122 002, Haryana, India

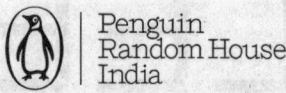

Penguin
Random House
India

First published in Ebury Press by Penguin Random House India 2016

ISBN 9788184006872

Typeset in Sabon by Manipal Digital Systems, Manipal
Printed at Repro India Limited

www.penguin.co.in

MIX
Paper from
responsible sources
FSC® C047271

To my family and patients who made this happen

CONTENTS

FOREWORD

Sleep is a fundamental state of life. It forms one-third of our existence. Even though the investigation into sleep goes back several thousands of years, we are still studying and learning new things about it today.

Modern sleep research is often considered to have started in the 1950s, with the monitoring of the sleeping brain and the description of three different states of alertness, by a group of pioneers, in the US and France. In the US, Azerinski and Dement, under the supervision of their professor, Kleitman, studied sleep at the University of Chicago, and in France, Michel Jouvet at the Universite de Lyon did the same. All three of them described the different sleep states based on the monitoring of brain-waves, eye movements and muscle tone of sleeping individuals.

Based on these initial descriptions, much research has been done that allowed an understanding of the fundamental role of sleep and the development of 'sleep medicine'.

Before this research, who would have believed we become paralysed about every 100 minutes during sleep, that we avoid consuming a lot of energy in our muscles, and that we redistribute our blood and all its nutrients toward our brain to perform critical intellectual tasks, allowing learning and memorization of the important facts of the day, improving our cognition during these segments of our sleep, and that we simultaneously prepare our brain to function at its best the next day?

It is now known that the controls of many vital functions are different during the two sleep states compared to wakefulness and that dysfunctions of these controls may occur only during sleep, and that investigating the health of a subject only during wakefulness may not be sufficient—some disorders may began during sleep and 'spill-over' during wakefulness, when many dysfunctions are well established.

Universities and schools of learning now have programmes investigating sleep, its many functions and pathologies. However, we are still in the developing stage in many areas with regard to this subject. If PhD programs involving sleep research are found in mathematical and physics departments, bio-engineering and business schools, and if medical schools have divisions of 'sleep medicine', this is still an exciting, new field that will further develop in many directions.

It is important that everybody has knowledge of where the field of sleep research and sleep medicine stands, and to provide the community the latest information on this field—we all experience sleep, sometime it is hurt by our activities and absence of knowledge, and we may suffer from its dysfunctions.

Dr Manvir Bhatia has been directly following the evolution of the field. She has participated in the study of normal sleep and she has cared for patients with sleep disorders, and knows first-hand the latest discoveries in sleep research and sleep medicine. Who would be more qualified than her to report where the field stands, where it is going and what are the latest developments.

I have known her for years, having met her at international congresses and at more research-oriented meetings, where the latest discoveries were presented. In this book, she has succeeded in presenting all the exciting new findings involving our sleep and its pathologies in a very articulate way. Often scientists are too close to their crops and do not know how to translate the field and its exciting discoveries to the community at large, but Manvir Bhatia has avoided these traps and has written a book that everybody will enjoy. The book also responds to questions that many of us have on the 'mysteries of sleep'.

Christian Guilleminault
DM, MD, DBiol.
Professor, Stanford University School
of Medicine, Division of Sleep Medicine

INTRODUCTION

I wanted to be a doctor for as long as I can remember. My desire to practice medicine was so strong that I did not even consider any other career. And when I began studying at the Christian Medical College, Ludhiana, I knew I was on the right track. My training focussed on patient care, and I learned to listen with empathy. This is one of the most important skills in my current practice, where I help patients with a variety of problems, especially sleep disorders. In order to help someone with a problem so personal, it is crucial to listen attentively to what they are saying.

After completing college, I chose to specialize in neurology, and began working with patients suffering epilepsy, at the All India Institute of Medical Sciences (AIIMS), Delhi. This project required patients to be monitored on video for prolonged periods of time, and I began noticing that while my patients slept, unusual events often occurred. Some would make bizarre movements in their sleep, while others would scream, attempt to hit objects around them, get off the bed and try to run, and so on. I could not clearly define or categorize these events, and so, motivated by the prospect of helping these patients, I began my journey into sleep medicine.

My journey began in 1995, when sleep medicine was still in its infancy in India. Therefore, to pursue my goal, I went to Harvard University, Boston, where I spent months preforming night duties, recording sleep and interpreting the data, participating in case discussions, becoming part of professional bodies on sleep medicine, and attending international conferences to satisfy my quench to learn more. I returned to India with the realization that there were still many things about sleep that the global medical community did not understand, and a renewed desire to continue my investigations.

Since then, I have made it a priority to conduct research and participate in the global dialogue on sleep by attending meetings and conferences on the subject. The more time I spend delving into this field, the more mysterious it becomes. We understand and accept now that sleep is one leg in the tripod of health, along with food and exercise. Each patient I treat provides me with a new perspective on the mystery of sleep, and improved technology continues to advance our knowledge on the mechanisms of sleep—what keeps people awake, and even the function of sleep.

After more than twenty years of working in the field, it is time for me to share what I have learned. In this book, I would like to discuss my understanding of how important sleep really is. My goal is the same as it has always been: to help as many people as possible, to improve their lives by improving their sleeping habits.

I hope that this book will clarify issues and fill in the knowledge gaps for those who want to know more about sleep, and ultimately, be used as a tool to help people live healthier happier and more productive lives.

WHY THIS BOOK?

We all have, at some point in our lives, experienced some issue related to sleep. Whether we suffer from chronic insomnia or simply feel less energetic than we would like to during the day, sleep problems deeply influence our lives. They manifest themselves as difficulty in falling asleep, the desire to sleep during the day, tiredness upon waking up, or persistent yawning. Whatever your sleep problem might be, this book will help you deal with it.

Here, I will describe sleep problems and their solutions in a way that everyone can relate to them—by including true stories of my patients and the actual ways in which we solved their problems. The first step towards resolving your sleep issues once and for all is to understand what actually happens in our bodies and brains when we fall asleep. I will explain this process in a way that will be comprehensible to all readers; I will also explain how to take your sleep quality into your own hands.

By the end of this book, you will understand the complexities of sleep and will be able to use this knowledge to change your life. I will touch upon how many hours of sleep an individual needs and how to control wakefulness. The aim of this book is to serve as an all-encompassing guide to sleep-related issues for everyone, regardless of age or gender.

We all know how difficult it is to function normally after a poor night's sleep. This book will unravel the multidimensional role of sleep in our lives. Read on . . .

TAKE A SLEEP TEST

1. Are you a loud, habitual snorer?
2. Do you have choking/difficulty in breathing at night?
3. Do you regularly feel tired, even after waking up from a full night's sleep?
4. Do you fall asleep while reading, driving or at home during the day?
5. Are you satisfied with your sleep?
6. Do you have difficulty in falling asleep?
7. Do you take sleeping pills?
8. Do you have difficulty in maintaining your weight?
9. Do you have pain in your legs upon lying down?
10. Do you have to go to the bathroom frequently at night?
11. Do you have high blood pressure/diabetes?

If you have answered 'yes' to two or more questions, it could be a symptom of a sleep disorder.

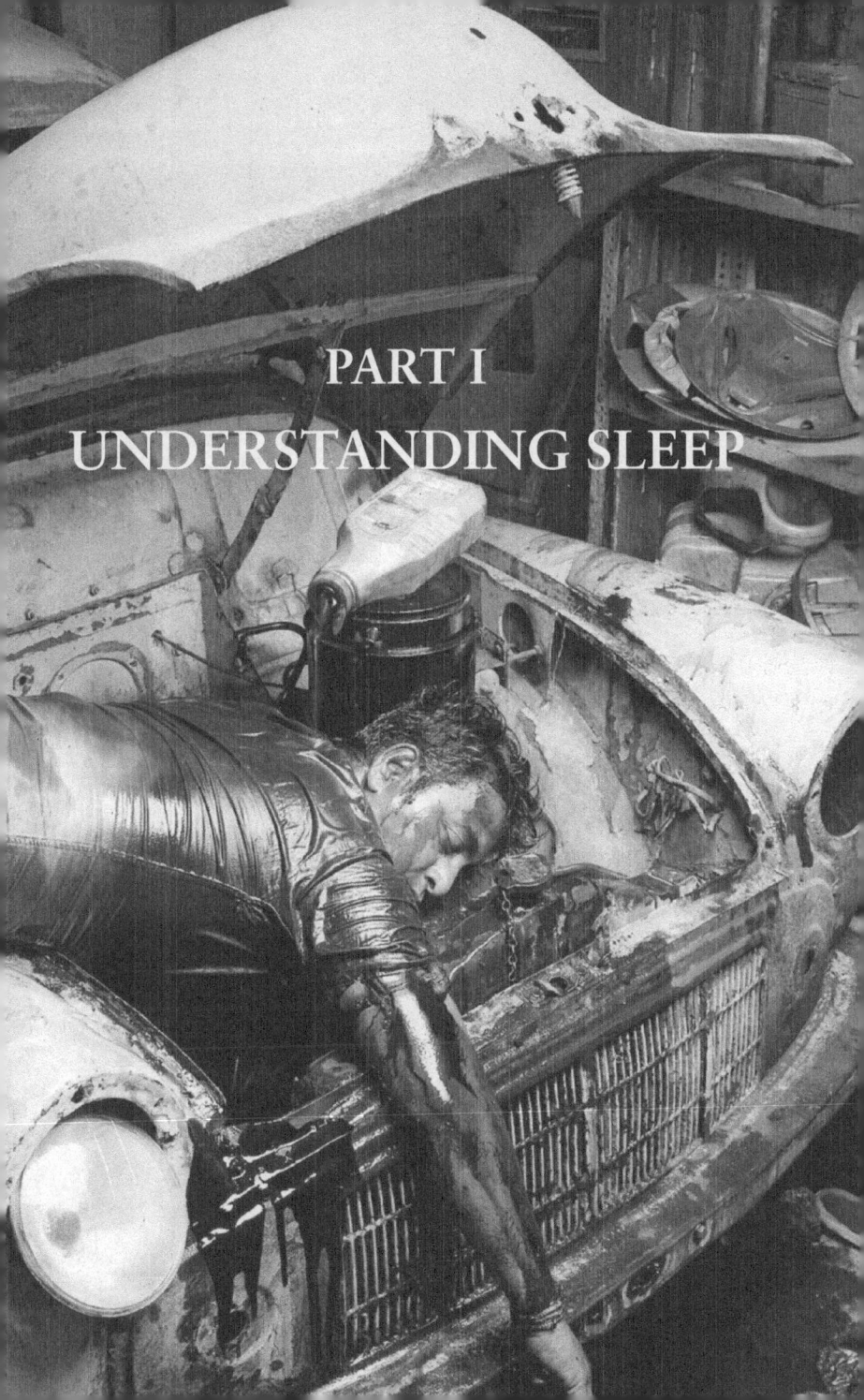

PART I
UNDERSTANDING SLEEP

1

WHAT IS SLEEP?

Here's a nugget of information to make you sit up and take notice. Did you know that the single biggest factor behind your success (or failure) is a five-letter word? Sleep.

Sleep is one thing that human beings all over the world share in common—regardless of age, gender, class or status. All of us sleep. Yet how many of us think about *why* we sleep? Even if, and when, we do think about it, sleep means different things to each of us. For some of us, sleep is a mystery; for some it is a memory booster; for others, it is a natural beauty treatment, and so on. For many, sleep is an enemy—a waste of time, a luxury. Everyone seems to have their own definition of sleep and the role they think it has in their lives. But, surely, there is universal agreement on the fact that sleep is an essential requirement. With so many varying personal definitions, what then is sleep?

The Oxford English Dictionary defines sleep as 'a condition of body and mind which typically recurs for several hours every night, in which the nervous system is inactive, the eyes closed, the postural muscles relaxed, and consciousness practically suspended'. As a sleep specialist, I disagree with this definition, as there is ample evidence now that the nervous system is far from inactive during sleep. What happens inside our body when we sleep? Brain imaging studies have proved and highlighted the fact that many areas of the brain become functional or show increased 'firing', or activity, during different stages of sleep.

A slightly more scientific definition can be found in Stedman's Medical Dictionary: 'A natural periodic state of rest for the mind and body, in which the eyes usually close and consciousness is completely or partially lost, so that there is a decrease in bodily movement and responsiveness to external stimuli.'

This focus on sleep is nothing new. Sleep has been a topic of interest for authors, poets, philosophers, priests and others for centuries now. Sleep has been mentioned in various, and very interesting, contexts in the ancient scriptures like the Vedas and the Ramayana, and, generally, in the Hindu mythology. It also finds mention in the Bible.

Today, though most people do not understand or think too deeply about why one sleeps, everyone has experienced the repercussions of a bad night's sleep. It tends to affect one's mood, concentration and attitude, and creates difficulties in problem solving. According to the Centre for Disease Control and Prevention, in USA, 'insufficient sleep is an epidemic'.[1]

It is linked to vehicle crashes, industrial disasters and chronic diseases such as hypertension and diabetes. On the other hand, the feeling of well-being after a good night's rest cannot be expressed fully. This is corroborated by statements made by people after successful treatment of their sleep problems. For example, a patient called the day after his treatment 'a bright, sunny day' as compared to all the days that had been 'cloudy and dull' prior to treatment. One patient said it was like a 'veil being lifted, a curtain being raised', while another patient said it was like wearing spectacles—you don't realize what you're missing unless it is treated.

Multidimensional Role of Sleep

It is important to understand why sleep is essential to human existence, even though some people consider sleep to be an enemy—probably because while sleeping, one does not engage in activities such as eating, working, etc. However, it is an acknowledged fact that sleep is a universal phenomenon and has been so since the beginning of existence. It has been observed that most animals and birds follow different sleeping patterns and positions. Horses need two–four hours of sleep, and usually sleep while standing; humans need an average of seven to eight hours of sleep, and prefer to lie on their backs. Some animals like bears go into hibernation for months and prefer to sleep on their stomachs. Therefore, one can assert, on the basis of the latest findings and the direction of ongoing research, that a majority of living beings, creatures and organisms require sleep.

For years, sleep was thought to be a passive process, when the brain and other functions simply shut down. Research over the last few years has proven this to be totally wrong. Given the essential nature and obvious importance of sleep for every living being on earth, it is vital to understand what constitutes sleep, why one sleeps, and the multidimensional role of sleep in living and leading a healthy life.

Key Points for Better Sleep

- Sleep is an essential requirement for all living beings.
- Many areas of the brain become functional or show increased activity during different stages of sleep.
- A bad night tends to negatively affect one's mood, concentration and attitude, and creates difficulties in problem solving.
- A good night's sleep imparts a distinct, highly beneficial feeling of well-being.
- It is vital to understand what constitutes sleep and why one sleeps.

2

WHY DO WE SLEEP?

For centuries, it was believed that sleep was merely a passive state in which the body and mind rested. Or, as Aristotle believed, sleep was just an unremarkable and unimportant period, marked by the absence of our usual sense of perception. But over the years, this concept has undergone a massive change with psychoanalysts like Sigmund Freud exploring sleep and the dimensions it opens up through the generation of dreams. His work has been significant in altering the dominant view on dreams. Through dreams, Freud sought to explore what he called the 'subconscious', which he believed held answers to people's behaviour and actions.

Although this book does not connect directly with Freud and his theory on dreams, it is an exploration of sleep, an attempt to understand the nature and importance of sleep, and its basic function.

We need sleep to keep us healthy, happy and ensure we are doing our best. Sleep is an active state important for renewing our mental and physical health each day. We can be our best selves when we get enough good sleep.

Your brain needs sleep, so you can:	Your body needs sleep, so your:
• Remember what you learn	• Muscles, bones and skin can grow
• Pay attention and concentrate	• Muscles, skin and other parts can fix injuries
• Solve problems and think of new ideas	• Body can stay healthy and fight sickness

Before we proceed any further, it is necessary for us to extend our discussion to understand why we sleep. At this juncture, it is important to share some research conducted on sleep and some of the theories constructed on why we sleep.

Energy Conservation Theory

While there is complete agreement that sleep is not a passive but an active process, and that it is an essential physiological process for humans and for most animals, numerous, and varied, theories exist on why this is so. One of these theories is the Energy Conservation Theory, according to which sleep acts to reduce the 'wear and tear' of the brain and to conserve energy. Sleep acts like a recharge for a battery, says this theory.

Warm-blooded animals, in particular, use a lot of energy to maintain their body temperature during sleep. They have two zones of temperatures to maintain: their core temperature and their shell temperature. The core temperature in humans, of the abdominal, thoracic and cranial cavities—the vital organs—is maintained by the brain. The core temperature of warm-blooded animals is reduced by 1°C during sleep, so we use less energy to maintain our core temperature. This theory is supported by the fact that smaller animals have a higher metabolic rate and sleep longer, while cold-blooded animals (reptiles, fish, etc.) need lesser periods of sleep. However, energy conservation is not the main purpose of sleep.

Preservation and Protection Theory

The second one is called the Preservation and Protection Theory. According to this theory, animals' chances of survival in the wild are increased exponentially by sleeping, because during their sleeping hours, the animals ensure that they are safely hidden from any prowling predator. This is, however, not applicable to all species, especially humans, in the twenty-first century.

Physical Restoration Theory

The third theory concerns itself with physical restoration of the organism's body. This theory states that sleep is essential for 'housekeeping' purposes—for the maintenance of mental and physical health. Sleep helps in the integration of new memories and in the storage of long-term memory. It is also a time for the repair and consequent renewal of tissues and nerve cells, and the cleaning of neurotoxins from the brain.

Sleep and its Multiple Benefits

In a sleep deprivation experiment conducted on rats, it was observed that sleep deprivation manifested itself in the poor healing of wounds and the development of skin lesions. The rats were unable to maintain a stable body temperature and eventually succumbed to death because of sepsis or sheer exhaustion. Thus, we can see that sleep plays an important role in the healing of wounds and the strengthening of the immune system.

Decades ago, there existed a hypothesis that sleep was essential for the functioning of the brain. This was because sleep allows the brain to relax its synapses to memorize and retain information acquired during the day. The brain employs 80 per cent of its energy to sustain synaptic activity. This means that with such a large portion of the brain's work dedicated to its synaptic activity, its only method of relaxation is sleep. A prolonged deficiency of sleep leads to memory loss and other disorders.

It is interesting to note that the brain uses the period of sleep to not only consolidate new memories into its system, but also to deliberately delete the ones it does not deem important, so that room can be made for new memories. Neurons, the key functioning element of the brain, are continuously active during the time we sleep. Thus, it is clear that sleep performs the function of refreshing the body and mind. It is, however, important to also point out that this is not its only function.

Sleep is indispensable to our existence, as research conducted over the years has shown that deprivation of sleep can become a powerful tool of torture. Experiments on animals have shown that sleep deprivation can lead to insanity and death, thus making it an efficient tool of persecution. Lack of sleep makes one very vulnerable and completely breaks down one's defences—that may not be so easily broken down with the deprivation of food and water.

Sleep deprivation results in a person being in a bad mood and exercising poor judgment when it comes to making important decisions. The age-old phrase 'sleep on your problem' may after all be true as research has shown that sleep helps people discover novel solutions to complex problems. Sleep deprivation takes a toll on our memories because they are essentially formed and stored when the brain is 'asleep' or 'offline'.

Memories are not isolated compact objects but interconnected webs of information. During sleep, this web is updated by the addition of new memories, whose placement is done in a manner that they are accessible when called upon by the brain.

When you get enough sleep, you can:	Without enough sleep, you can:
Pay better attention while learning new things	Forget what you learned
Be creative and think of new ideas	Have trouble making good choices
Fight sickness so you stay healthy	Be grumpy and in a bad mood

(*Contd.*)

When you get enough sleep, you can:	Without enough sleep, you can:
Be in a good mood	Have trouble playing games and sports
Get along with friends and family	Be less patient with family and friends
Solve problems better	Have trouble listening to parents and teachers

Sleep psychologist Matt Walker says 'sleep is essential for learning'. The brain is like a sponge, which absorbs all the information and allows old and new memories to interconnect. Sleep is essential , and is the basis, for human creativity. 'Like good cooking it is not enough to chop up the ingredients and put them together. The brain needs time to let things marinate.'[1]

Therefore, it comes as no surprise that a lack of sleep—regardless of the cause, habits, lifestyle or sleeping disorders—will affect all the functions in a human's brain. The facts on record, some of which have been enumerated in this chapter, establish very clearly that sleep is a necessity and not a luxury, a friend and not an enemy. Gambling it away would not be a wise choice.

Key Points for Better Sleep

- Sleep is essential to form new memories, consolidate old ones and remove unnecessary ones.
- Sleep maintains and balances our moods, behaviour and emotions.

- Sleep fights infections.
- Sleep is essential for bodybuilding, growth and rejuvenation.
- Sleep helps to discover novel solutions to complex problems.

3

UNDERSTANDING SLEEP

Did you know that we are not in one constant state of sleep the whole night? It is divided into two parts, depending on the varying depths of sleep. There are recurring cycles of 90–110 minutes of two categories of sleep known as Non-rapid Eye Movement (NREM) and Rapid Eye Movement (REM). Through the night, there are a total of four or five cycles of sleep. The first part is NREM, which is followed by REM sleep. The amount of time spent in each stage changes through the cycles, which increase and decrease as the night progresses.

Why are the two categories of sleep called NREM and REM? REM sleep was first described in 1952 by two scientists: Eugene Aserinsky and Nathaniel Klietman. They observed patients in hospitals had irregular and jerky eye movements while asleep. On studying this phenomena further, they found that this happened at times and not throughout the sleep period.

Thus, the part of sleep with rapid eye movements was called REM sleep and the one without the movements was called NREM.

Further research over the years has elaborated on both stages and has also shown what happens to the body's functions, hormone secretions, etc., during the different stages of sleep.

Non-rapid Eye Movement

Stage 1 of NREM is also known as light sleep. We usually enter sleep in this stage, and are half awake and half asleep during this period.

In this stage, besides a decrease in muscle activity, one can:

- Occasionally hear a person talking
- Be awakened easily
- Feel an occasional muscle twitch

Stage 2, also known as true sleep, forms the largest chunk in time of our sleep.

We enter this stage about ten minutes after going to sleep. Our breathing and pulse rate slow down during this time. Typically, it is identified by the presence of sleep spindles. Measured while recording the electrical activity of the brain (EEG), sleep spindles consist of a rhythmic activity at 12–14 hz, shaped like a spindle— hence, the name. Sleep spindles are now thought to be correlated with memory.

In fact, alterations in sleep spindles are seen in certain psychiatric disorders.

Stage 3, also known as deep sleep, usually comes after forty–fifty minutes of falling asleep.

In this, breathing slows down further, the heart rate drops and muscle activity (tone) decreases. If awakened during this stage, it is difficult to adjust immediately to one's surroundings and a person can feel groggy and disoriented for some time. This state is also called 'sleep drunkenness'. Many disasters, accidents, etc. have been linked to it. Sleepwalking, night terrors and bedwetting are also seen during this stage.

This stage is important for memory consolidation, especially declarative memory.

Slow Wave Sleep

Deep sleep, or stage three of NREM sleep, is also called Slow Wave Sleep (SWS). SWS is the constructive phase of sleep, in which the mind and body can rebuild themselves. The growth hormone is secreted during this time to repair damaged tissues. Thus, a decrease in this stage of sleep results in the accumulation of harmful, toxic substances that can damage the brain and impair memory consolidation. During sleep, all metabolic processes are employed in 'building' organs and tissues, and new molecules are formed.

The REM cycle is important for procedural memory to retain information. Procedural memory is that part of our memory which is concerned with retaining information regarding procedures and processes of how to do things and perform certain actions. SWS is important for declarative memory— factual knowledge (general knowledge, vocabulary), and information attached to a specific event (episodes in one's life).

Experiments have shown that tasks learned during daytime are performed better the following day, when a person has had a good night's sleep. The experiments have also concluded that the same tasks cannot be performed when the person has not been allowed to sleep. This sleep cycle is concerned with weeding out and deleting information the brain does not deem important.

Rapid Eye Movement

Rapid Eye Movement is the state in which the eyes are constantly moving, hence the name. It constitutes about 20 per cent of the total sleep at night for an adult.

The first REM period occurs seventy to ninety minutes after a person falls asleep. There are usually three–four REM periods during the night. As the night progresses, the REM periods gradually get longer. This state has been described as 'an active brain in a paralysed body'. It is also associated with the occurrence of maximum number of dreams.

During REM, there is a rise in blood pressure (BP) and heart rate, with irregular respiration. This stage is important for procedural memory—knowledge of how to perform a task (how to drive a car, bicycle, etc.). Brain activity during REM sleep is similar to the brain activity one has in the waking state.

Thus, there is a constant variation in states between wakefulness, NREM and REM sleep throughout the night. Moreover, REM sleep is largely devoted to brain repair and restoration, while NREM sleep is when the body repairs and restores itself. To feel refreshed upon waking up, it is essential not only to have an adequate duration, i.e. seven–eight hours, of sleep, but also spend adequate time in each stage of sleep. If the duration of sleep is seven or eight hours but one is still tired, then the issue that has to be resolved is the quality of sleep. Eight hours of sleep also saves energy equal to the amount one gets after consuming a slice of toast. Thus, contrary to a certain theory, energy conservation is not the main purpose of sleep.

Sleep Increases Brain Connections

Studies have indicated that sleep is very important in the development of the brain, especially for babies. There is increased brain activity and this argument is supported by the fact that children spend a much longer portion of their time sleeping, unlike adults. REM sleep is particularly important for the development of the brain and a child's body spends almost 80 per cent of its time in the REM cycle. It has been mentioned earlier that sleep plays an important role in the consolidation of memory and the learning of new information. New neuronal pathways are re-enforced and cemented during sleep, which allow all of these processes to take place.

These neuronal pathways have been known to play a major role in memory consolidation and it's processing, before introducing and memorizing a new experience into the fold. Sleep helps in converting short-term memories to long-term memories and also works on the reconsolidation of the already existing long-term

memories. This process of addition and revision ensures
that no information is inaccessible to the brain.

Key Points for Better Sleep

- We are not in one constant state of sleep the whole
  night.
- Sleep is divided into parts, depending on the varying
  depths of sleep.
- There are two categories of sleep known as Non-
  Rapid Eye Movement (NREM) and Rapid Eye
  Movement (REM).
- REM sleep is devoted largely to brain repair and
  restoration, while NREM sleep is that time when the
  body repairs and restores itself.
- To feel refreshed upon waking up, it is essential not
  only to have an adequate duration, i.e. seven to eight
  hours, of sleep, but also spend adequate time in each
  stage of sleep.

4

HOW MUCH SLEEP DO WE NEED?

Have you ever wondered how much sleep do you really need? There is no simple answer to this since there is no fixed amount of time an individual should spend sleeping. An average adult needs seven–eight hours of sleep. However, individual sleep needs vary, particularly according to age, and are unique to each person. Some individuals are 'long sleepers' and require more than eight hours of sleep, while some are 'short sleepers'. This is usually a genetic predilection, which means an in-built body clock determines the amount of sleep that is required. For example, 6–10 per cent of adults need more sleep (nine–ten hours a night) than the average. About 5 per cent can manage with six hours and the remaining 85 per cent need seven–eight hours. Sleep is said to be adequate when you wake up refreshed, without an alarm clock, feel fresh throughout the day, with no daytime sleepiness. Sleep is said to be adequate when 'measured' not only in quantity (number of hours) but also quality (i.e. spending enough time in different stages of NREM and REM sleep).

HOW MUCH IS ENOUGH?

Age	Daily sleep requirement
Newborns (0–2 months)	12–18 hours
Infants (3–11 months)	14–15 hours
Toddlers (1–3 years)	12–14 hours
Pre-schoolers (3–5 years)	11–13 hours
Young children (5–10 years)	10–11 hours
Adolescents (10–17 years)	8.5–9.25 hours
Adults	7–9 hours

Sleep Requirements Keep Changing

According to the National Sleep Foundation, the single factor that affects sleep requirement is age. The make-up of our sleep in terms of NREM sleep and REM sleep changes throughout our lives (see diagram).

Age-related changes in total amount of sleep and REM Sleep

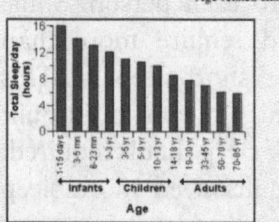 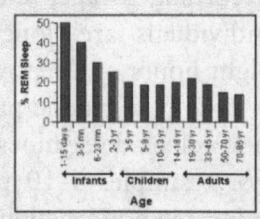

Babies, when born, sleep for almost twelve–eighteen hours a day and the majority of their sleep is REM sleep. The duration of sleep gradually decreases. School-going children need ten hours, adolescents nine hours, and adults need seven–eight hours of sleep. Along with the decrease in duration, the REM sleep percentage also decreases. The increased REM sleep in children could be due to the number of changes and the pace at which their brain develops at that age.

The control or timing of sleep is governed by a hormone called melatonin. This usually starts to rise at sunset, peaks a few hours later and then gradually decreases. However, during adolescence and teenage, there is a delayed release and peak of this, resulting in the delayed onset of sleep. This causes them to feel sleepy later than their usual time, around 11–12 p.m., and thus they experience difficulty in waking up early, especially for school. In fact, these children are prone to mood changes, irritability and often get labelled as ADHD (Attention Deficit Hyperactive Disorder). Numerous states in the US have kept this in mind and have pushed school timings back with excellent results. In these schools, not only did the children do well academically, but their behaviour also improved.

Ageing and Sleep

Older people also undergo changes in their sleep—both in duration, i.e. quantity, and stages of sleep, i.e. quality. Sleep, on the whole, is shorter, not very continuous and breaks more often (also called fragmented sleep). This is probably due to the change in the cells that control sleep. They undergo degeneration and cause a decrease in deep sleep and REM sleep. This results in complaints from older patients that they don't sleep well and wake up often during the night.

There is a higher percentage of time spent in light sleep or Stage 1 of NREM. This is why the elderly often complain of poor sleep. The reasons for this could be a host of health-related issues, including arthritis, respiratory disorders, sleep apnoea (an interruption in breathing during sleep caused by a narrowing of the breathing passage leading to partial or complete closure), restless leg syndrome and the like. Most of these go undiagnosed and untreated in older adults because they are considered a part of the process of aging. It is, however, important to address these issues as they are curable with treatment.

Key Points for Better Sleep

- An average adult needs seven–eight hours of sleep. However, individual sleep needs vary and are unique to each person.
- Sleep is said to be adequate when 'measured' not only in quantity (number of hours) but also quality (spending enough time in different stages of NREM and REM sleep).
- According to the National Sleep Foundation, the single factor that affects sleep requirement is age.
- The make-up of our sleep in terms of NREM and REM sleep changes throughout life.
- It is important to address sleep problems in elderly people as they are often curable with treatment.

5

EFFECTS OF SLEEP DEPRIVATION AND SLEEP DEBT

Today's fast-paced lifestyle affects our sleep cycle in a big way. Sleep deprivation results in direct implications on our body, such as an increase in the blood sugar level, high blood pressure and so on. Sleep is an active resting state essential for our mental, physical and emotional well-being. When one is deprived of sleep, the brain cannot function properly, which in turn affects reasoning, thinking, one's emotional state and judgement. According to the Harvard Medical School, sleeping for just five hours increases the risk of death from all causes by 15 per cent.[1] Sleep deprivation leaves one tired and exhausted, affecting concentration. This, naturally, affects decision making.

Sleep deprivation has many other ill effects:

- **Emotional impact:** Lack of sleep has a significant impact on our emotions, and our moods. Often, it results in mood swings, besides increasing irritability.

- **Mental health:** There is a bi-directional relationship between mental health and sleep deprivation. People with depression, bipolar disorder and schizophrenia can have altered sleep patterns. Sleep deprivation in those with existing mental health disorders can lead to the worsening of the illness. In fact, an extended period of sleep deprivation can trigger mania in people suffering from Manic Depressive Psychosis (MDP, also known as bipolar disorder), impulsive behaviour, depression and paranoia. There is also evidence that sleep deprivation precedes bipolar disorders and depression, thus making it important to detect this condition at its start and offer intervention.

- **Micro sleep:** Sleep deprivation can result in micro sleep, resulting in tragic accidents involving aeroplanes and nuclear reactor accidents. (Micro sleep comes in brief spurts, which occur spontaneously and are uncontrollable).

- **Weakened immune system:** During sleep, protective cytokines (molecules which stimulate the movement of cells towards sites of inflammation, infection and trauma), infection-fighting antibodies and cells are produced. These fight with bacteria and viruses to protect us. Sleep deprivation impairs our body's ability to fight infection and thus, it also takes longer for the body to recover from an illness.

- **Weight gain:** Sleep deprivation is also reported as a risk factor for weight gain. Less than five hours of sleep is associated with a 50 per cent chance of being obese. There is an increased production of the stress hormone, called cortisol, and a decrease in the level of leptin, the satiety hormone, which leads one to eat more. Accompanying this is an increase in the level of ghrelin, an appetite stimulant, which then causes increased secretion of insulin which promotes fat storage.

- **Cardiovascular system:** Sleep deprivation results in an increase in blood pressure and causes changes in the lining of arteries. This leads to an increased risk of heart disease due to weight gain and also adverse changes in the arteries.

Symptoms of Sleep Deprivation

How can you tell if you are sleep deprived? Sometimes the signs can be difficult to notice as they are very subtle, but generally you can tell if you are:

- Irritable on waking up
- Have difficulty in getting out of bed in the morning
- There is increased tiredness during the day
- There is a desire to take an afternoon nap

If you are chronically sleep deprived, you may not even recognize the symptoms. It's somewhat like viewing the world when you have impaired vision—you cannot experience the difference unless you try on glasses.

SLEEP DEBT

Sleep debt or sleep deficit is a situation where one gets less sleep than the amount one's body needs. For instance, if you need eight hours of sleep but get only six hours per night, there is a debt of two hours, and if it is carried out on five days, then the total debt is 5x2 = 10 hours.

This is something like a bank debt that we owe our body; it results in changes in our emotional, physical and mental behaviour.

Eventually, the body will require this debt be repaid, which it is does by catching up on sleep. This is called recovery sleep. However, the recovery sleep required is not equivalent to the sleep loss; it needs to be approximately three times more. For example, if you have a sleep debt of two hours, you need approximately five–six hours of sleep to make up the loss, and not two hours of sleep.

Sleep debt can be short term or long term. If it is chronic, or long term, it is known to cause serious conditions, such as diabetes, obesity, stroke, heart attacks, immune changes and high blood pressure. This also causes changes in mood, resulting in depression and bipolar disorder.

There is a change in the hormones that control appetite and satiety, gherlin and leptin, respectively, causing overeating, weight gain, insulin resistance and an increased risk of type 2 diabetes.

Lack of sleep or increased wakefulness causes an increase in stress hormones, or cortisol. This causes a rise in blood pressure. In fact, recent research has suggested that poor sleep can cause changes in the deposition of substance amyloid beta that results in memory disorders, dementia and Alzheimer's disease.

Less sleep has also been shown to increase the risk of cancer. A large study shows that women who sleep for more than nine hours a day have a lower risk of breast cancer than those who sleep for less than nine hours.

It has been widely observed that sleep debt that occurs in shift workers can make them more prone to accidents and injuries. The risk of accidents is higher on the night shift, especially if a larger number of night duties are done together. Major disasters, such as Chernobyl and the Bhopal gas tragedy, have occurred at night and lack of sleep has been implicated as a factor in them.

According to a study, 'Road traffic accidents, are another major source of concern with sleep loss. It has been seen that majority of road traffic accidents occur at 2–3 a.m. (which is related to the sleepiest time in our cycle). In the USA, the National Highway Safety Administration estimates that falling asleep while driving is responsible for around 100,000 accidents each year in the USA alone, including 71,000 injuries and over 1500 deaths. It has been estimated that 17 hours of sustained wakefulness (for example, from 7 a.m. until 12 midnight) leads to a decrease in performance equivalent to a blood alcohol level of 0.05% (two glasses of wine), the legal drink driving limit in many countries.'[2]

Nowadays, the mean sleeping time is estimated to be approximately seven hours, suggesting a reduction of around an hour's sleeping time compared with fifty years ago. In a study conducted in Finland, '20.4% of participants were found to have insufficient sleep. In Japan, a study of 4000 adults revealed that 28% had fewer than 6 hours of sleep on weekdays. These studies point to a high rate of insufficient sleep in developed countries'.[3]

Laws Governing Sleep-deprived Driving

Driving when sleep deprived can cause serious safety hazards. There are various laws that govern driving and sleep. According to a study, 'In the European Union, drivers' working hours are regulated by an EU regulation which entered into force on April 11, 2007. The non-stop driving time may not exceed 4.5 hours. After 4.5 hours of driving, the driver must take a break period of at least 45 minutes. However, this can be split into 2 breaks, the first being at least 15 minutes and the second being at least 30 minutes in length.'[4] One is allowed a daily driving time limit of nine hours in total, which can be extended to ten hours around twice a week, not more. Taking this into account, the weekly driving time limit is fifty-six hours.

A report on understanding pilot fatigue states that cargo pilots, on the other hand, are required to have a minimum of ten hours of rest in between shifts, out of which eight hours should be uninterrupted sleep. The report states that 'pilots will be limited to flying eight or nine hours, depending on their start times. They must also have 30 consecutive hours of rest each week, a 25% increase over previous requirements.'[5]

The DGCA has also laid down rules and regulations for Indian pilots to ensure safety and prevent pilot fatigue.

INSOMNIA

ARE YOU AN INSOMNIAC?

A good night's sleep is as important to your health as diet and exercise. So if you are having trouble sleeping, it's important to talk to your doctor. Your sleeplessness could be what's called insomnia. The word insomnia comes from the Latin words *in* (no) and *somnus* (sleep). It literally means 'no sleep' or inability to sleep. Insomnia is an experience of inadequate or poor quality of sleep, usually seen with one or more of the following complaints:

- Difficulty falling sleep
- Difficulty staying asleep
- Waking up too early in the morning
- Having sleep that is non-refreshing

Due to the stressful lifestyles these days, most people experience a bout of insomnia at some point in their lives.

Insomnia is a symptom of another problem, much like a fever or a stomach ache. It may be caused by a number of factors.

I Lifestyle

a) Stimulants: Caffeine keeps people awake as it stays in the bloodstream for six hours. So, an evening cup of tea or coffee may disturb your sleep.

b) Nicotine: This makes it difficult for you to fall asleep.

c) Alcohol: You may think that having a glass of wine at bedtime will help you sleep. But while it may help you fall asleep quickly, alcohol is likely to make you wake up frequently throughout the night.

d) Work hours: If you are a shift worker, you are more likely to experience sleep problems.

e) Poor habits: Working on the Internet till late at night may also disrupt your sleep. Watching TV just before you sleep, especially disturbing events and horror movies, can also interfere with sound sleep.

f) Exercise: Regular exercise helps people sleep better. The best time to exercise is the afternoon. Do not exercise close to bedtime.

II Psychological Factors

a) Tendency towards insomnia: Some people are more likely to develop insomnia when stressed out.

b) Persistent stress: Relationship problems, a child with serious illness or an unrewarding job may contribute to sleep problems.

c) Psycho physiological (learned) insomnia: Constant worry about sleep, trying very hard to sleep, makes it worse.

III Environmental Factors

a) Noise: Keeping the bedroom as quiet as possible can aid in sleeping well.
b) Light: Light can disrupt your sleep. Use shades or heavy curtains to keep the bedroom dark.

IV Psychiatric Illness

a) Patients suffering from depression and anxiety also suffer from poor sleep.

V Primary Sleep Disorders

a) Sleep-related breathing disorders: People with snoring and choking in sleep—Obstructive Sleep Apnoea (OSA)— wake up frequently at night.
b) Restless legs syndrome: Pain, discomfort on lying in bed, with a desire to move the legs, and relief of discomfort on movement, causes difficulty in falling asleep.
c) Periodic limb movements: These are brief muscle contractions which may cause leg jerks that last a second or two. This results in a brief interruption of sleep.

VI Medical Factors

a) Complaint of poor sleep can develop as a result of several types of medical problems. Physical discomfort from conditions as diverse as fever, body pains, arthritis, cough, breathlessness, post surgery and going to the bathroom frequently at night can all lead to disturbed sleep.

Signs and Symptoms: How to Identify Insomnia?

Daytime Symptoms: Feeling tired throughout the day; feeling fatigued, irritable or sleepy, and having poor concentration or attention.
Night-time Symptoms: Difficulty falling asleep, difficulty staying asleep, frequently waking up during sleep or waking up too early in the morning.

When to Seek Medical Help?

It's time to seek help if your sleep has been disturbed for more than two weeks and interferes with the way you feel or function during the day.

Celebrities and Sleep

Modern-day life boasts of lifestyles so exhausting that sleeping is considered a waste of time. But for celebrities, who are more than familiar with night life, sleep remains an essential desire of their lives that they have to constantly neglect.

In an article in the NY Daily News, Nicole Lyn Pesce wrote, 'Throughout history, powerful and influential figures from politicians to performers, inventors to artists have carried out incredible acts on very little sleep. It begs the question: Does needing a lot of sleep, rather than a little, separate the great from the rest of us? You can rest easy: there is no magic number when it comes to getting enough sleep. As it turns out, different people function better by sleeping on different schedules.' The writer pointed out that 'Leonardo da Vinci may have created the Mona Lisa on two hours of sleep a day, broken up into fifteen-minute naps every four hours—but Albert Einstein took 10 hours of sleep each night, as well as daytime naps!'[5]

Inventor Thomas Edison slept for just four or five hours a night and thought sleep was a waste of time. His light bulb has been helping students and workers burn the midnight oil ever since.

But when it comes to the celebrities' sleeping habits, however, there's usually more than meets the eye. Edison may have been dismissive of sleep, but he often napped a lot during the day. Winston Churchill, Ronald Reagan, John F. Kennedy and Napoleon also took forty winks in the afternoon to make up for their late nights.

From the point of view of sleep, Winston Churchill is the most famous narcoleptic. Narcolepsy is a neurological disorder and a narcoleptic brain does not have the ability to regulate sleep–wake cycles normally. Narcoleptics experience bouts of extreme daytime sleepiness and have sudden uncontrollable urges to sleep that can come about at any point in time.

From starring in *Sleepless in Seattle* to being sleep deprived, Tom Hanks recently talked about the anxieties he experiences when he doesn't catch enough Zs. Many celebrities have constantly emphasized the essential role that sleep plays in living a healthy and productive life.

Closer home, B-town beauty Deepika Padukone, who is known for her radiant glow, also talks about the effect of sleep on one's skin, going as far as saying that 'lack of sleep accelerates the aging process' and affects your regular fitness. According to fitness fanatic Sonam Kapoor, not getting enough sleep can harm your body, as it will not get the time to recover from stress, and will consequently affect your workout and long-term fitness. Her father, Anil Kapoor, holds a similar perception as he emphasizes that sleep relaxes and refreshes your mind. At the end of the day, it is more important to be mentally fit than physically fit.

What is the solution to beating the many ill effects of sleep deprivation? Simple! Just make sure you get enough sleep. There will be guaranteed improvement in the quality of your waking life, your mental sharpness, productivity, emotional balance, creativity, physical vitality and maintaining an ideal weight. No other activity delivers so many benefits with so little effort.

Key Points for Better Sleep

- When you are deprived of sleep, the brain cannot function properly, which in turn affects reasoning, thinking, one's emotional state and judgement, and often causes accidents.
- Sleep deprivation is also reported as a risk factor for weight gain. Less than five hours of sleep is associated with a 50 per cent chance of being obese.
- Sleep deprivation leads to an increased risk of heart disease due to weight gain and also adverse changes in arteries.
- Sleep deprivation, or insufficient sleep, leads to sleep debt (also called sleep deficit), which has to be repaid through what is called recovery sleep.
- Recovery sleep is not equivalent to the sleep loss, but needs to be approximately three times more.

6

CAN SLEEP BE MEASURED?

Yes, sleep can be measured—just like blood pressure, blood sugar, cholesterol, etc. But why is measuring sleep important? It is important because it enables you to empower yourself with the knowledge to judge your condition or problem, it tells you how you can benefit yourself, and how you can avoid harm to yourself and others. Measuring sleep can be especially useful for those in high risk professions. In several countries, there are laws which specify and govern the amount of sleep required for drivers, pilots, etc. There are two ways of measuring sleep—subjective and objective.

Subjective Means

Sleep can be measured by subjective means (i.e. the individual does a self-assessment).This is a set of questions you answer to decide if there's any sleep-related issue.

The subjective tests are a set of questions, which, when placed together, have the potential to identify individuals with sleep problems and they can be then evaluated further. Some of the tests are the STOP-BANG Scoring Model, the Epworth Sleepiness Scale (see visuals), etc.

STOP-BANG Scoring Model[1]

The STOP-BANG model is a questionnaire used to identify obstructive sleep apnoea. This can be used by the patient themselves and also by doctors as an initial screening tool. There are a total of eight questions with choices 'Yes' or 'No'. The questions are easy to remember and start with the 'alphabets', for instance:

S = Snoring (Is your snoring loud and disturbing?)
T = Tired (Do you feel sleepy during the day?)
O = Observed (Has anyone observed that you stop breathing/start choking during sleep?)
P = Blood Pressure (Are you being treated for high blood pressure?)
B = BMI (Is your body mass index >35kg/m2?)
A = Age (Is your age> 50 years?)
N = Neck size (Is your neck size >17 inches for males and >16 inches for females?)
G = Gender (Are you a male?)

One point is given for every 'Yes'. The maximum score is eight and the scores of:

0–2 = low risk
3–4 = intermediate risk
5–8 = is high risk for OSA

The Epworth Sleepiness Scale[2]

The Epworth Sleepiness Scale (ESS) is a simple tool that comprises a set of questions to gauge the subject's sleepiness in a few situations. This was developed by Dr John Murray in 1991. There are a total of eight questions, where an appropriate number assesses the subject's chances of dozing off in a given situation:

0 = never doze off
1 = slight chance of dozing off
2 = moderate chance of dozing off
3 = high chance of dozing off

The situations include activities such as sitting and reading, watching TV, sitting inactive in a public place, as a passenger in a car, while talking, resting after lunch (lying and sitting) and if the car stops at a traffic for few minutes.

The total maximum score is 8 questions x 3 = 24.

One can calculate your own score to assess the sleepiness. This questionnaire has been tested and researched extensively, and score <10 is considered to be normal, 10–16 suggests increased daytime sleepiness, and >16 is suggestive of being dangerously sleepy.

Thus for scores >10, you should meet a sleep specialist to determine the cause of this daytime sleepiness.

Berlin Questionnaire[3]

The Berlin Questionnaire is a validated screening tool to measure the risk of Obstructive Sleep Apnoea (OSA) in the general adult population and various high-risk population groups. Developed in 1988 in Berlin, Germany, this questionnaire has been a popular tool to classify a patient as 'high risk' or 'low risk' for OSA. There are nine simple questions, based on three domains:

1) Details of snoring during sleep
2) Daytime sleepiness and fatigue
3) Presence of obesity or hypertension (risk factors for OSA)

A person positive for two or more domains is considered to be at 'high risk' for sleep apnoea based on the Berlin Questionnaire.

In the first domain of the Berlin Questionnaire, questions related to snoring are asked. They help judge the presence, frequency and loudness of snoring. Snoring is a consistent feature present in most sleep apnoea patients and considering it the other way around, it is believed that half of all snorers have sleep apnoea. Snoring is also the most common reason why patients visit sleep clinics. In this domain, questions about a bed partner-witnessed stoppage of breath at night is also asked, which is considered more specifically related to sleep apnoea than many other symptoms. In fact, the technical definition of sleep apnoea itself incorporates 'a ten second or more of a pause in breath', which means this stoppage of breath only which is confirmed polysomnographically.

The second domain deals with the daytime symptoms of sleep apnoea—fatigue and sleepiness during daytime and a sense of non-refreshing sleep in the morning. Daytime symptoms of sleep apnoea are present in around 50 per cent of sleep apnoea patients; hence, these questions.

The third, and final, domain tries to screen for sleep apnoea through two strongly associated risk factors— hypertension and obesity. Obesity is defined as presence of a BMI>30. A BMI of thirty was taken considering the German population while formulating the questionnaire and validating it. For the popularity that the Berlin Questionnaire has received as a screening tool, there have been attempts to further modify it to make it more sensitive, and specific for different ethnicities and races. The modified Berlin Questionnaire is a tool developed in AIIMS, New Delhi, which has been shown to have a similar sensitivity and specificity, but with far fewer trials to display its consistency and accuracy. It simply takes a lower threshold for obesity (twenty-five instead of thirty) in the third domain.

To be considered positive for each domain, a patient needs to have positive answer to at least two questions each in domain one (snoring) and domain two (daytime features). For domain 3, presence of either hypertension or obesity is considered a positive response. The final score is 'high risk' for sleep apnoea if at least any two of these three domains are positive. Anyone not satisfying the above categorization will be considered low risk for sleep apnea. 'High risk' patients should then ideally undergo a sleep study to diagnose OSA or to refute its diagnosis. The sensitivity and specificity of Berlin Questionnaire has been tested on various populations and geographic distributions.

Pittsburgh Sleep Quality Index (PSQI)[4]

PSQI is a questionnaire with twenty-four questions on sleep which help determine the quality of sleep in a person and classify him/her as a 'healthy sleeper' or a 'poor sleeper'. The set of twenty-four PQSI questions cover the seven components of sleep: subjective sleep quality, sleep latency, sleep duration, habitual sleep efficiency, sleep disturbances, use of sleeping medications and daytime dysfunction seen over the preceding thirty days. Each component is scored in an ordinal scale of 0–3. Finally, a global PSQI score is also calculated summing up the individual components.

The first component, subjective sleep quality, is judged based on the overall quality of sleep in the preceding thirty days. The answer is recorded on a ordinal scale of 0 to 3, where 3 means 'very bad' to overall sleep quality and 0 meaning very good sleep quality, with 1 and 2 given to intermediary quality of sleep.

The second component measured is sleep latency. This is the time one takes to go into sleep after lying down in bed and switching off the lights. A longer sleep latency is suggestive of a poor sleep quality, therefore given more points, while a latency of <15 minutes is considered normal in this scale.

The third component is a measure of total sleeping time. Longer hours score fewer points, while shorter time spent sleeping score more in this component.

The fourth component measures the sleep efficiency, which is the percentage of time one spends sleeping against the total time spent in bed. A value above 85 per cent is normal and gets a score of 0, while sleep efficiency of <65 per cent gets a score of 3; other values fall in the middle.

The fifth component is a different kind of measure to look into the various causes that disturb sleep, like pains, nocturia, temperature problems, bad dreams and so on. The number of times each problem disturbs sleep are summed up and graded. The greater the disturbance, the higher the score.

The sixth component measures an individual's extent of dependency on sleeping pills to get some sleep. In this component, the number of nights a person uses sleeping pills is taken into account to grade the severity of the condition. Ideally, the information is incomplete without the type, amount and duration of the drugs used, but since it's a simple screening tool, it serves its purpose well.

The seventh component is a measure of daytime sleepiness/fatigue of a person as it asks about the number of days when a person has been sleepy or has dozed off in inappropriate places. The severity is again graded in a scale of 0–3, with a higher score meaning a greater number of days were spent dozing off, which is a measure of night-time sleep deprivation manifesting in the day.

A Global PSI Score of >5 is considered to have a sensitivity of 89.6 per cent and a specificity of 86.5 per cent to understand a sleep problem. Therefore, a person with such score should then visit a sleep specialist or his physician.

Sleep Diary

A sleep diary is a sheet, which is filled by the subject about activities carried out during the day and night. The person is instructed to enter the time of consuming food or caffeine, exercise, medications and the time spent in bed, for daytime naps and at night. This provides useful information about activity during the day in bed, sleep, etc. This can be recorded by the individual for 1–2 weeks and gives insight into the individual's activities and how to improve his/her lifestyle. It also helps if the subject is being treated by a physician and is advised about improving sleep.

TWO WEEK SLEEP DIARY

INSTRUCTIONS:
1.   Write the date, day of the week, and type of day: Work, School, Day Off, or Vacation.
2.   Put the letter "C" in the box when you have coffee, cola or tea. Put "M" when you take any medicine. Put "A" when you drink alcohol. Put "E" when you exercise.
3.   Put a line (I) to show when you go to bed. Shade in the box that shows when you think you fell asleep.
4.   Shade in all the boxes that show when you are asleep at night or when you take a nap during the day.
5.   Leave boxes unshaded to show when you wake up at night and when you are awake during the day.

SAMPLE ENTRY BELOW: On a Monday when I worked, I jogged on my lunch break at 1 PM, had a glass of wine with dinner at 6 PM, fell asleep watching TV from 7 to 8 PM, went to bed at 10:30 PM, fell asleep around Midnight, woke up and couldn't got back to sleep at about 4 AM, went back to sleep from 5 to 7 AM, and had coffee and medicine at 7:00 in the morning.

Today's Date	Day of the week	Type of Day Work, School, Off, Vacation	Noon	1PM	2	3	4	5	6PM	7	8	9	10	11PM	Midnight	1AM	2	3	4	5	6AM	7	8	9	10	11AM
sample	Mon.	Work	E						A					I								C M				
18/2/10	Thurs	Vacation	T M						T	E				I												
19/2/10	Fri	"									M			I										T	M	
20/2/10	Sat	"												I												
21/2/10	Sun	"	T M		C				T	E	C		m	I												
22/2/10	Mon	"																								T m

Objective Means

There are objective means as well (standardized laboratory tests) to measure sleep. Sleep can be measured objectively by recording activity from the brain, muscles, eye movements, breathing, snoring, oxygen saturations, EKG, body position, leg movements, etc. through the night.

Sleep Study Test

Sleep study is an overnight test to record information from various positions of the body, which is then analysed. This is done using sensors placed on various parts of the body— data is collected and then evaluated later to understand normal and abnormal functions. The normal functions include brain activity, along with recording of eyes and muscles to provide information about the quality and quantity of sleep, normal breathing patterns, the oxygen saturation throughout the night, with body position, the EKG for the whole night and variations in heart rate. The abnormalities can be seen in the poor quantity and quality of sleep, snoring, pauses in breathing (apnoeas), oxygen drops during the night, increased muscle activity, and/or electrocardiogram (ECG) abnormalities.

There are numerous types of applications available for measuring sleep (see page 123 for more details). Sleepbot, for example, tracks sleep and motions during sleep. A few gadgets are also available for monitoring sleep talking/sound recording, etc. However, the majority of apps available help you sleep soundly rather than measuring sleep.

Key Points for Better Sleep

- It is important to measure sleep because it enables you to empower yourself with knowledge to judge your condition or problem and that of others.
- Sleep can be measured by subjective means (i.e. the individual does a self-assessment).
- There are objective means as well (standardized laboratory tests) to measure sleep.
- Tests can provide specific information about the quantity (duration) of sleep and quality of sleep.
- There are numerous types of applications as well for sleep, but most of them help you get sound sleep rather than measuring sleep.

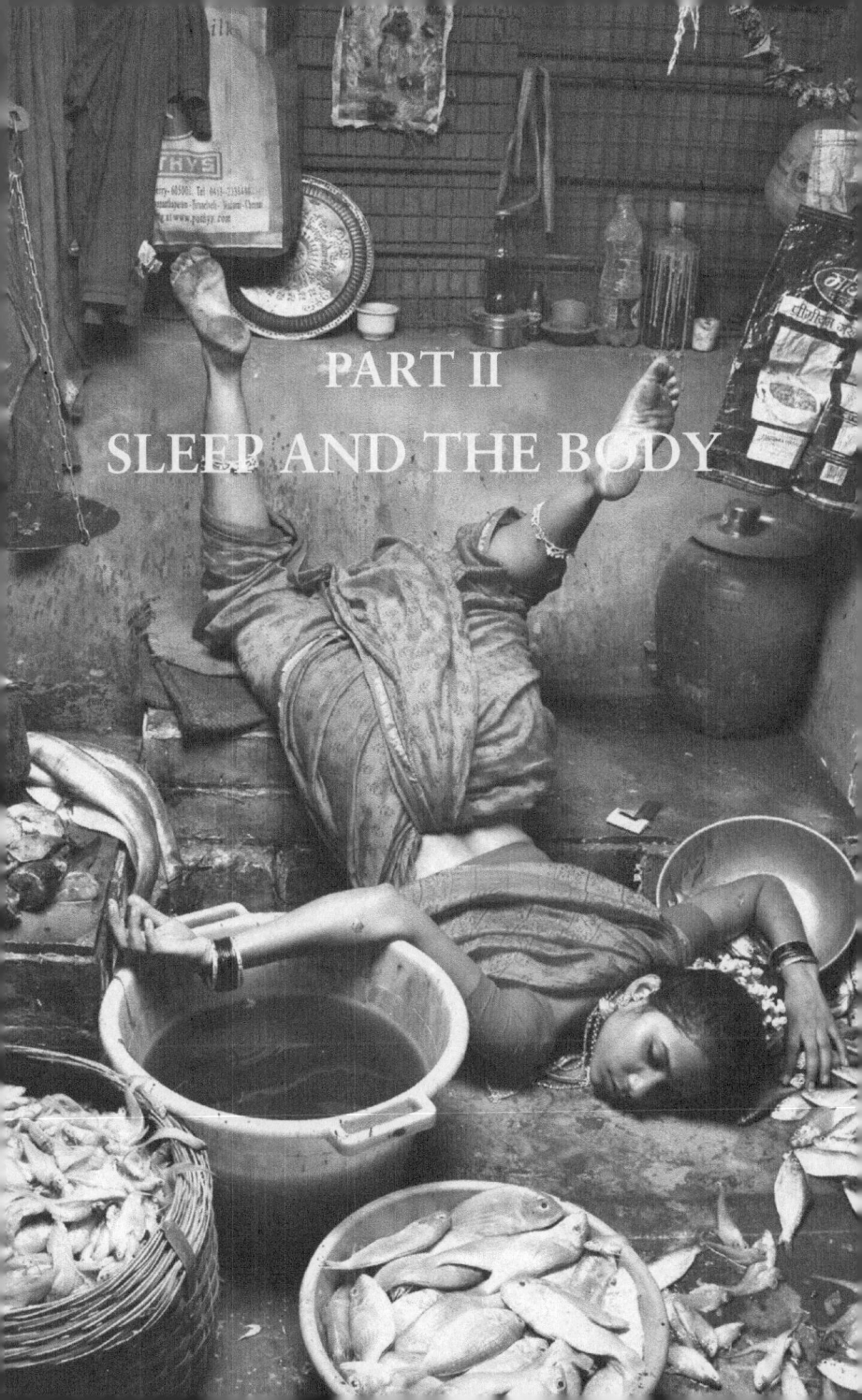

PART II

SLEEP AND THE BODY

7

SLEEP AND HEALTH

Major disasters, such as the world's worst nuclear disaster at the Chernobyl power plant in Ukraine, the Bhopal gas tragedy, several oil spills, the Challenger Explosion in the year 1986 (a major space shuttle disaster that killed all seven crew members) have all been linked to sleep deprivation resulting in loss of vigilance and, consequently, poor judgment. Over the years, various studies have shown that approximately 100,000 accidents occur per year are due to the drivers' sleep deprivation. Other studies have shown the percentage of accidents that occur as a result of sleepiness is around 20 per cent.

This goes to show that there is a clear association between sleep and traffic accidents. Generally, accidents caused by drowsiness and falling asleep are the result of drivers being unable to control the brakes or steering due to their impaired state. The tragic Mangalore air crash on 22 May 2010 was also attributed to poor judgement as the pilot woke up from slow wave sleep and was unable to gauge the landing conditions. A major disaster in the New York subway, in 2014, was also sleep related. It was later revealed that the driver of the train that derailed was suffering from a serious sleep disorder. Because of the sleep link, drivers are now increasingly being tested for sleep disorders. If investigated properly, it may be found that countless accidents in which the cause was not determined could have been due to sleep-related issues.

The fact is, sleep is a basic necessity of life—as important to our health and well-being as air, food and water. When we sleep well, we wake up feeling refreshed, alert and ready to face challenges. In our daily lives, too, sleep has an impact on many areas. If there are sleep problems, our jobs, relationships, productivity, health and safety (and that of those around us) are all put at risk. Research suggests that sleep loss may be on the rise due to changes in self-reported sleep duration over the last fifty years.

In 1960, 'a survey of over 1 million people found a modal sleep duration of 8.0–8.9 hours. In 2000, 2001 and 2002, polls conducted by the National Sleep Foundation indicated that the average duration of sleep for Americans had fallen to 6.9–7.0 hours. Overall, sleep duration thus appears to have decreased by 1.5–2 hours during the second half of the 20th century. Today, many people are in bed only 5–6 hours per night on a regular basis.'[1]

The Endocrine System and Sleep

Effects of Partial Sleep Loss

Real life situations of chronic partial sleep loss appear to be much more common now. Recently, a few studies have examined the impact of this new reality on hormones, the metabolism and immune functions. The earliest study measured hormonal and metabolic parameters in subjects studied after six days of sleep restriction (four-hour bedtimes) and after full sleep recovery (six days of twelve-hour bedtimes). Later on, studies were done to evaluate the impact of less severe sleep restriction (6.5 hours per night) over one week, as well as the effects of short-term sleep curtailment (two days with four-hour vs twelve-hour bedtime).

Partial sleep loss is seen to cause a rise in the stress hormone, cortisol. Continued sleep loss or chronic sleep loss causes cortisol to further rise, which can result in the development of insulin resistance, obesity and diabetes. Another hormone that is affected is the thyroid stimulating hormone (also known as thyrotropin or TSH), which decreases, resulting in poor functioning of the thyroid. The good news is that this recovers when sleep is improved.

Another important hormone, the growth hormone (GH), is also altered by sleep loss. It can cause growth impairment in children.

Impact of Sleep Loss on Hormones Controlling Appetite

Sleeping and feeding are intricately related. There are two hormones which are principally involved in food and our eating behaviour. Gherlin is secreted by the stomach and stimulates appetite. Sleep loss results in an increase in gherlin, causing increased hunger and appetite, especially for carbohydrate-rich, starchy food, such as cakes, pastries, pasta, pizza, etc. Does this sound familiar to those who have unexpected hunger pangs at night?

Leptin is the hormone released by fat cells. It sends a message of satiety to the brain (stop eating, in simple terms). This hormone markedly decreases with sleep loss.

Thus, this combination of a decrease in leptin and an increase in gherlin results in an increased calorie intake and weight gain.

The interesting corollary is that in current times, the incidence of obesity is doubling and this is a mirror image of the general decrease in sleep duration, thus proving that sleep loss is a cause of obesity.

An analysis of the link between sleep duration and obesity among adults notes that 'short sleep duration was significantly associated with incidence of obesity, whereas long sleep duration had no effect on future obesity among adults...Sleep is probably not the only answer to the obesity pandemic, but its effect should be taken seriously, as even small changes in energy balance are beneficial.'[2]

Metabolic Implications of Recurrent Sleep Curtailment

We have already discussed the effect of hormones on the glucose metabolism. Sleep loss is associated with increased risk of type 2 diabetes. This is due to glucose intolerance, i.e. the ability to metabolize glucose is impaired in those with sleep loss.

Research has shown that normal healthy individuals have higher morning blood sugar levels with six days of sleep restriction (four hours in bed). This is further confirmed by intravenous glucose tolerance testing. Thus, sleep restriction of even less than one week can result in a pre-diabetic state.

This could be due to the effect of sleep loss on various mechanisms responsible for glucose metabolism. There is an increase in cortisol, increased sympathetic activity and changes in the secretion of the growth hormone.

You may do a host of things to remain healthy, but unless you ensure good quality and adequate quantity of sleep, those things will not hold much weight.

Key Points for Better Sleep

- Elevations of evening cortisol levels in chronic sleep loss are likely to promote the development of insulin resistance, a risk factor for obesity and diabetes.
- Thyroid function can be markedly altered by partial recurrent sleep loss.
- Sleep loss is associated with an increase in appetite that is excessive in relation to the caloric demands of extended wakefulness.
- The regulation of leptin, a hormone released by the fat cells that signals satiety to the brain and thus suppresses appetite, is markedly dependent on sleep duration.
- Sleep loss could be a risk factor not only for accidents but also for major chronic diseases.

8

SLEEP AND BEAUTY

For years, beauty and sleep have been considered to be in a directly proportional relationship (remember Sleeping Beauty?). You don't require a medical degree to link sleep with beauty, as the effect of the former on the latter has always been quite apparent. Despite the obvious time-honoured results, the younger generation has often thoughtlessly disturbed their biological clock and ignored the scientific relevance of good sleep. In any case, there are many fads and myths which need to be debunked, and reality needs to be placed in its correct perspective through factual data related to sleep and beauty.

The Science behind Sleep and Beauty

Dr Doris J. Day, author of *Forget the Facelift*, says: 'Your skin, and your whole body, goes into repair mode when you sleep.' While you sleep, your skin renews itself. New skin cells grow and replace older cells. 'It's repairing and restoring and rebalancing,' Day writes.[1] The effects of poor sleep is not just restricted to the skin but goes on to give rise to a lot of diseases. Many doctors say that good sleep reflects on the face instantly—in the form of freshness and radiance of the skin. This is because the protein and collagen formation in sleep (which give the face a natural facelift and glow) is double at night compared to daytime.

While we are sleeping, a lot of metabolic and hormonal changes happen in the body, which can be disrupted due to improper sleep.

Effects of Improper Sleep on Skin

- **Impairs collagen production:** Improper sleep affects skin function and utility, and impairs collagen production. Collagen is very useful in protecting the skin against ultraviolet rays and it provides firmness to the skin. It also protects the skin against bacterial infections, seals in moisture, improves elasticity and preserves its youthful, healthy appearance.
- **Causes premature ageing of the skin:** 'When you're tired, blood doesn't flow efficiently,' says Michael Breus, MD, author of *Beauty Sleep*.[2] A continued lack of sleep or disturbed sleep patterns can give rise to puffy eyes, lacklustre skin and can even result in the premature ageing of the skin.
- **Can break down skin collagen:** Cortisol is arguably the most important of the glucocorticoids and there is evidence that our body releases more of this 'stress hormone' when it is sleep deprived. In excess

amounts, cortisol can break down skin collagen, the protein that keeps skin smooth and elastic.

- **Affects beauty maintenance:** Having understood the importance of collagen, one more fact that we need to understand is that the upkeep of skin is not dependent on medical or cosmetic care, but on the lifestyle we follow. If something as simple as sleep holds great significance in maintaining our beauty, why not capitalize on it?

- **Impedes the release of growth hormone:** While we are sleeping, the growth hormone is released, which helps increase muscle mass, thickens skin and strengthens bones.

- **Affects overall health:** It is important to keep in mind that beauty is not only about the face. It is about the whole body and one's overall health. Health is affected because of poor sleep, which, in turn, takes a toll on the body and eventually on the face. It is often said that the face is a mirror to the health of a person, and it would be right to add that health is a mirror to the sleeping pattern of a person and vice versa.

- **Accelerates the ageing process:** In humans, sleep debt and stress can trigger inflammatory skin conditions such as eczema and psoriasis. An article on how beautiful skin begins with a good night's sleep states that sleep debt 'can also exacerbate both atopic dermatitis and irritant contact dermatitis. Scientists attribute the link between chronic insomnia and skin disorders to the immune-altering effects induced by the release of excess glucocorticoids triggered by sleep debt and stress. This class of hormones regulates the metabolism of glucose. Every cell in the human body possesses receptors for glucocorticoids, which play a crucial role in immune function. Excess glucocorticoid production has been shown to negatively affect nearly every tissue in the body and accelerate the ageing process.'[3]

More Advantages and Disadvantages

The advantages of good sleep are not the only measuring rod to estimate the correlation between beauty and sleep. Stating the hazards and disadvantages can also serve the purpose.

Insufficient sleep disturbs the functioning of the outermost layer of the skin, which is called the stratum corneum. As a result, the skin is unable to recover from daily injuries. The stratum corneum serves two main functions:

- Prevents foreign microorganisms from getting into the skin
- Locks in moisture

Besides these two important functions, the significance of the stratum corneum is the fact that it contains keratin, which keeps the skin hydrated. Due to improper sleep, adequate moisture is not retained in the skin. Insufficient sleep thus adversely affects the skin barrier's ability to do its job. This in turn can cause dehydration, which can make fine lines more noticeable. It is a common fact that moisture helps plump up the skin, while the lack of moisture can make your skin droop, making it feel like a deflated balloon.

An article in the *Huffington Post* states that 'Poor sleep can lead to increased stress hormones in the body that increase the severity of inflammatory skin conditions such as acne or psoriasis,' explains Jessica Krant, MD, MPH, assistant clinical professor of dermatology at SUNY Downstate Medical Center and founder of Art of Dermatology in New York.[4] This can result in increased itching, which can disrupt sleep. 'While you're sleeping, the body's hydration re-balances. Skin is able to recover moisture, while excess water in general in the body is processed for removal. Not getting enough sleep results in poor water balance, leading to puffy bags under your eyes and under-eye circles, as well as dryness and more visible wrinkles.'[5]

Undeniable Benefits of A Good Sleep

Sleep and beauty are interconnected, and it is not possible to escape the after-effects of poor sleep. These facts are undeniable. Briefly, the power of good sleep and the benefits it yields can be enumerated as follows:

- A good night's sleep helps in strengthening the immune system, which ensures that infections are fought and injuries are repaired.
- Eight hours of undisturbed sleep can work wonders on one's skin because while we sleep, protein is made in our skin which protects the skin against ultraviolet radiation.
- Proper sleep also helps in burning calories.
- A good night's sleep keeps a person happy and saves him/her from mood swings. 'Positivity leads to beauty'—this is something we all know as true.

- Adequate sleep is conducive to collagen and growth hormone production, which eventually benefits the skin by helping it maintain its glow and radiance.
- A good sleep regulates the metabolic rate, which helps increase the replenishing of fresh cells on the surface of the skin.
- People who enjoy a good night's rest can avail of natural anti-ageing benefits!

Does Lack of Sleep Cause Dark Circles?

'Lack of sleep causes blood vessels to dilate, causing the look of dark circles,' says dermatologist Sonia Badreshia-Bansal, MD, University of California, San Francisco.[6]

However, insufficient sleep is not the sole reason behind dark circles. Many other factors, for instance genetic ones, might have a role to play in it. But lack of sleep makes the blood vessels under the skin more apparent. Decreased blood circulation might worsen the problem and leaves the face looking tired. Insufficient sleep contributes to puffiness under the eyes and eye bags.

Simple Steps to Ensure Good Beauty Sleep

Follow these simple steps for a good beauty sleep:

- If possible, bathe before going to sleep.
- Make sure the pillow is comfortable.
- Take special care of the bed sheets and pillow covers. If they are soft and comfortable, then you are most likely to enjoy a good night's rest.

- Avoid consumption of coffee three–four hours before sleeping.

How Much Sleep is Enough?

After reading all the data-based positive and negative points listed in this chapter, beauty freaks should not think that sleeping for ten–twelve hours will enhance their looks tremendously. The hazards of excessive sleep are tantamount to that of poor sleep. Experts agree unanimously that six–eight hours of sleep is ideal for almost every individual.

Key Points for Better Sleep

- The protein and collagen formation in sleep (which gives a natural face lift and glow) is double at night, when compared to daytime.
- While we are sleeping, a lot of metabolic and hormonal changes happen in the body, which can be disrupted due to lack of sleep.
- Not getting enough sleep can lead to dehydration of the skin, which, in turn, makes fine lines more noticeable.
- Sleep-deprived individuals appear less healthy, more tired and less attractive than those who have received a full night's sleep.
- Insufficient sleep plays a role in causing puffiness under the eyes and eye bags.

9

SLEEP AND FOOD

Sleep and food are two of the most basic and essential components of a healthy body. They affect the body in many ways, and must be balanced with care and knowledge to promote a healthy and long life. There are many popular sayings about sleep and food, like 'don't sleep immediately after eating', 'don't drink coffee before sleeping' or 'eat light food when you wake up'. When it comes to health, one encounters so much information every day that it becomes important to separate facts from fiction. Only then can we practice what will truly yield results.

Author Michael A. Grandner, psychiatry instructor and member of the Center for Sleep and Circadian Neurobiology at the University of Pennsylvania, researched the ways an individual's sleep depends on their nutritional intake. Grandner and his colleagues found that 'calorie intake varied across the groups, with short sleepers consuming the most calories, followed by normal sleepers, followed by very short sleepers, followed by long sleepers. When they looked at food variety, they found this was highest in the normal sleep group and lowest in the very short sleep group.'[1]

How Poor Sleep affects Diet

Lack of adequate sleep is connected to the desire to consume artificial sugar, carbohydrates and fats in excess. While a person who has had a proper night's sleep is found to have more regular and balanced eating habits, inadequate sleep increases the appetite, causing people to feel hungry as soon as they wake up. An analysis showed that, compared to the diet of the normal sleep group, 'Very short sleep was linked to less intake of tap water, lycopene (present in foods that are red and orange in colour, for instance tomatoes) and total carbohydrates. Short sleep was linked to lower intake of vitamin C, tap water, selenium (found in nuts, shell fish and meat) and higher intake of lutein/zeaxanthin (found in green, leafy vegetables). Long sleep was tied to lower intake of choline (found in eggs and fatty meats), theobromine (present in chocolate and tea), dodecanoic acid (a saturated fat) and total carbohydrates, and a higher intake of alcohol.'[2]

These links remained even when other factors that might explain this relationship, such as demographics, socio-economics, physical activity and obesity, were taken into account.

Soporific Foods

Soporific foods are those that induce sleep.

Yogurt, milk, cheese, oats, bananas, poultry, eggs, peanuts and **tuna** all aid sleep because they contain the amino acid tryptophan, which, when combined with calcium and magnesium, helps the brain manufacture the sleep-inducing substance melatonin.

Almonds contain both trytophan and calcium, and are a rich sleep-inducing food.

Cheese also contains tryptophan, which has been shown to reduce stress and induce sleep. So cheese may actually help you have a good night's sleep.

Honey signals the brain to turn off orexin, a neurotransmitter linked to alertness. Overall, honey has a soothing effect on the body.

Potatoes induce sleep by eliminating acid, which can interfere with tryptophan.

Turkey is loaded with tryptophan and acts as a great soporific agent.

Chamomile prepared in the form of tea is a very effective cure for insomnia. To make it even more effective, add a few drops of honey.

Bananas contain potassium and magnesium, which, as stated earlier, contribute greatly to healthy sleep.

Oatmeal contains high amounts of melatonin, leading to good sleep.

Food that Keeps Us Awake

Caffeine has an awakening effect on the body. It tightens the muscles to ready them for action and causes the liver to release sugar into the bloodstream for extra energy.

Alcohol affects REM sleep time and often leads to waking throughout the night. In a study of twenty-seven men and women, between the ages of twenty-one and twenty-six, it was shown that people who drank alcohol took longer to fall asleep.

Tomato-based products cause acid reflux and heartburn, which prevent a good night's sleep.

High fat food like French fries and potato chips not only increase the fat in the body but also don't let a person fall asleep.

Cured meats like bacon, sausages and pepperoni contain high levels of tyramine, an amino acid that boosts the secretion of the brain stimulant norepinephrine, which keeps a person awake.

Aged cheese also contains the amino acid tyramine, which is believed to keep people up late.

It is thus important to work out a diet that will contribute to a good night's sleep. This is especially important in today's fast-paced world, where picking up a quick meal and skipping balanced meals and consuming too much junk food and canned food, have become the norm rather than the exception. What was said at the beginning of this chapter also encompasses the cardinal concluding principle: sleep and food are two of the most basic yet essential components of a healthy body, with good sleep being dependent on a balanced diet.

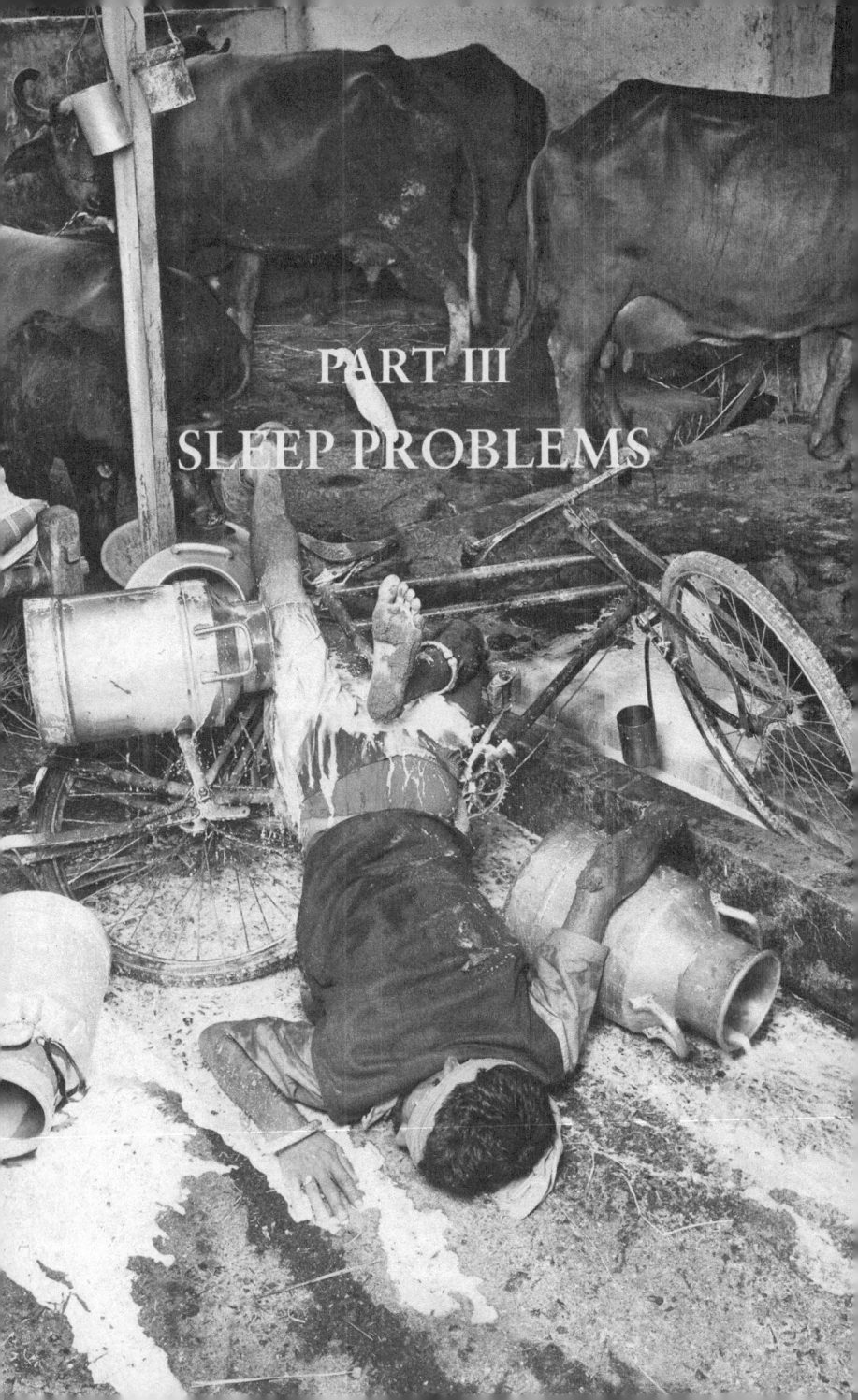

PART III

SLEEP PROBLEMS

10

COMMON SLEEP DISORDERS

Y ou'll be surprised to know that there are more than eighty types of sleep disorders. An estimated 50–70 million US adults have sleep or wakefulness disorders, and an estimated 150 million adults across the developing world suffer from sleep related problems.[1] However, the most common complaints I hear are of one feeling very sleepy, the inability to fall asleep or abnormal behaviour in sleep.

In the following chapter, I shall describe a few common cases related to sleep that came to me and how they were tackled.

EXCESSIVE SLEEPINESS

'Oh! I feel very sleepy all the time.' This is a common complaint heard from many people these days. Curiously, people who can't sleep are never able to imagine that the other extreme can also occur, and vice versa. However, both problems—of feeling sleep and not being able to sleep—are seen frequently. Both problems have their roots in what controls wakefulness and sleep, which has already been discussed in Part 1 of this book. Understandably, both problems have a major impact on the lives of those affected by them.

Case Study

A twenty-seven-year-old girl, a marketing consultant, came to meet me one day. She had been suffering from excessive daytime sleepiness for approximately five–six years. When I made her go down the memory lane, she admitted that she had always had trouble waking up for school and used to miss her bus very often. She could never attend her 9 a.m. classes in college despite adequate sleep at night. Somehow, she pulled along. But now the sleepiness was causing her great distress and embarrassment, and was interfering with her career, her relationship with her family and boyfriend.

She had also become very irritable, and preferred to be alone and avoided social gatherings. Her usual bed time was between 12–1 a.m., but was she was unable to wake up before 10 a.m., and was thus late for work every day. Her office began at 10 a.m., but after taking the metro train, she reached office only at 11.30 a.m. For the past few months, she had also been feeling extremely tired and sleepy during the day, and kept yawning constantly. The sleepiness was very severe while she was driving. In fact, she very nearly had an accident once. The car went off the road for a few seconds as she'd probably dozed off. She stopped driving after that day. In office, she tended to doze off during office conference calls and while working on the computer. She had gained 9–10 kg in eight months. She also disclosed that she had very vivid dreams, especially early in the morning.

She said she also found herself shivering and occasionally stammering when appearing for an interview. On being prompted, she recalled suffering from shivering

---

Sleep Study

Poly-somnography, also called sleep study, is an overnight test used to diagnose sleep disorders. The test records your brain waves, the oxygen levels in your blood, heart rate and breathing, as well as eye and leg movements during sleep.

---

in the legs during debates, etc. in school. Her family history, too, showed major sleep problems. Her father, aged fifty-nine years, had died in his sleep. He had been obese and also had a snoring problem (OSA: obesity + snoring problem). Her two elder siblings, though, were fine.

Medical investigation showed she had decreased vitamin D, vitamin B12 and iron levels. These, however, did not explain her increased sleepiness. To discover the cause, we conducted an overnight sleep study (for quantity, quality of sleep, and to determine the percentage of time in each stage of sleep and the time taken to fall asleep).

This was followed by a daytime test used to measure her excessive need to sleep. Both the tests were abnormal. The night test clearly showed that she was able to fall asleep within five minutes of going to bed and there was also an increase in the REM sleep component; in fact, she entered REM sleep in three naps during the day. These were conclusive of a disorder called narcolepsy.

Narcolepsy

Narcolepsy is a condition where there is a severe deficiency of the wakefulness promoting neurotransmitter called orexin. This deficiency results in severe sleepiness, with REM sleep intruding into the day, causing cataplexy—shivering and stammering during emotional excitement. This is a chronic condition, often with a lag period to the tune of five–fifteen years between the symptoms and diagnosis. People suffering from this condition are said to be lazy, depressed, with low motivation, etc. It is not understood that this is an organic problem, and should be tackled accordingly and appropriately. Here is the solution to it:

General Lifestyle Changes

• Maintain a regular time for waking up and going to bed.
• If very sleepy, take a short nap, and avoid driving or any task which can lead to injuries.
• Maintain healthy food habits and an exercise programme.
• Take planned naps if very sleepy.

Medication

• The patient was given stimulants, which helped keep her awake during the day.

What Could be Done to Improve her Quality of Life?

There is medication available to keep one awake; these are called stimulants.

The patient was prescribed medicines to decrease her REM sleep. REM is an active stage of sleep where we do most of our active dreaming. Our eyes actually move back and forth during this stage, which is why it is called Rapid Eye Movement sleep. This promotes wakefulness during the day, along with measures to take structured naps during the day. These take away the drive for sleep and the person can stay awake for longer periods.

NARCOLEPSY WITH CATAPLEXY

Let's look at another category of sleep problems. The person seeking a solution, a class XII student, said, 'Oh! I wish I was more alert! I don't think anyone can imagine what I go through. The day is a nightmare; I constantly feel like taking a nap. I have become the subject of jokes among classmates and family friends, not to mention school teachers.' This is the story of a seventeen-year-old girl. She can recall always being sleepy, with difficulty in staying awake.

Case Study

'There was huge uproar in the house every morning, with my family trying to wake me up for school. Then the fight continued within me to stay awake while my brain kept shutting down. The classes were a nightmare with information seeping in only intermittently. At other times, I went blank. As you can imagine, the final contents did not make any sense. Very often I was found napping, with my head on the desk, without me even realizing when I put my head down. I would find myself being woken up by the teacher or my classmates, and found that I had become an object of jokes and laughter in the classroom.

'Desperate to stay awake, I discovered my own antidote to it—a mechanism to handle this sleepiness. I started chewing gum—which became a persistent habit—to the point of my jaw hurting.

'The second problem was that I found myself on the floor a few times while listening to a joke being related by friends; initially not only my friends but I, too, was surprised to see myself on the floor. Then I learned to sit if I was relating or listening to a joke. When I described this to my doctor, Dr Manvir Bhatia, I was told that this condition is called cataplexy.

'The surprising thing was that I found myself far away, in la-la land, even during the short naps I had in class—I was having vivid dreams.

'Here goes my day:

6 a.m.: The alarm rings . . . rings . . . and rings . . . Half awake, I press the "snooze" button and go back to dreamland.

7 a.m.: Mom, busy preparing my tiffin, shouts from the kitchen to get me out of my slumber, but to no luck.

7.30 a.m.: Finally, I get out of bed, freshen up and rush to school.

8 a.m.–2 p.m.: It's sheer torture trying to concentrate, take notes and stay awake. I nod off frequently and hit my head on the desk, and feel as if my brain is shutting down.

'I am back home at 2 p.m. Post lunch, I take a long nap, and am unable to get up till 5 p.m. I have to be woken up and dragged outside for a walk. Then I'm home again, do some homework etc., have dinner at 8 p.m., and am asleep by 8.30 p.m. The night is full of nightmares, and I constantly wake up feeling extremely hungry. This leads to frequent trips to the refrigerator. All this led to a weight gain of 15 kg.

'Let's discuss the other harrowing symptoms—my mood and behaviour. I became very irritable, got angry at the smallest things, snapped at my mother very often. So I met a sleep doctor; honestly, I didn't think something like that existed. Dr Bhatia asked me to share my day and night routine and then suggested I get a complete sleep study done, to understand the sleep patterns, quality of sleep and quantity of sleep. This was followed by a daytime test called MSLT.'

MULTIPLE SLEEP LATENCY TEST

The Multiple Sleep Latency Test (MSLT) is a sleep disorder diagnostic tool. It is used to measure the time elapsed from the start of a daytime nap period to the first signs of sleep, called sleep latency. The test is based on the idea that the sleepier people are, the faster they will fall asleep.

The tests revealed an increased sleep drive and were highly suggestive of narcolepsy. As I said earlier, this is a condition with a severe deficiency of the wakefulness-promoting and sleep-stabilizing chemical, orexin. Besides sleep, orexin also influences appetite, metabolism, etc., resulting in mood changes and obesity. There is a significantly shortened sleep latency (i.e. the person very rapidly enters sleep) with increase in duration of REM sleep and sleep fragmentation or interrupted sleep. Daytime is also distressing for people suffering from this problem as they tend to fall asleep in all kinds of situations—when busy and also when sitting idle. This was demonstrated in the daytime test, which revealed that the patient could fall asleep very quickly when given an opportunity to do so.

What Could be Done to Improve Her Quality of Life?

The patient was prescribed stimulants to decrease her REM sleep and promote wakefulness during the day, along with measures to take structured naps during the day. Today, according to the patient, 'I am studying in college after completing my class XII, thanks to Dr Manvir Bhatia. In fact, I am now president of the theatre society and have a large number of friends.'

Key Points for Better Sleep

- General lifestyle changes along with medication, both preferably suggested by a sleep specialist, will definitely result in better sleep.
- Maintain a regular time for waking up and going to bed.
- If very sleepy, take a short nap, and avoid driving or any task which can lead to injuries.
- Maintain healthy food habits and an exercise programme.
- Can also take planned naps if very sleepy very often.

SHIFT WORK ISSUES

Does shift work, a common part of life these days, affect one's sleep? Though the concept of working at night and sleeping during the day no longer raises eyebrows, working in shifts can be stressful for a person. Let's see how.

Case Study

'I am twenty-five-year-old, working in an international firm, living in India, doing a night shift to match the time zones abroad, 9 p.m. to 6 a.m. On reaching home at 7 a.m., I relax for a while, watch TV, have some food, spend time on the phone, surf the Internet, etc., and then try to get some sleep. Here begins the struggle. My body is extremely tired, but I simply cannot fall asleep. I wait and wait, hoping sleep will come, but no such luck. My brain is racing with thoughts which have no sense or connection with the current day. Tick-tock . . . the clock ticks away and soon the household wakes up.

'I keep lying in bed, hoping for some luck with sleep. Sometimes I manage to doze off for a few hours, but feel very un-refreshed, tired, irritable and disturbed by the slightest noise around. I finally get out of bed at 3 p.m., grab a bite, and am in bed again waiting for sleep. Then, I get out of bed at 6 p.m. grab a Red Bull to make me feel alert, and it serves its purpose.

The office vehicle comes to pick me up at 8 p.m., and then I head out to work, not, as you can imagine, in the best of moods or with enough physical energy.'

What Does Shift Work Do?

Shift work acts against the body clock and the circadian rhythm—a roughly twenty-four hour cycle in the physiological processes of living beings, including plants, animals, fungi and cyanobacteria. Circadian rhythms are endogenously generated, although they can be modulated by external cues, such as sunlight and temperature.

Sleep is regulated by two body systems: sleep/wake homeostasis and the circadian biological clock. When we have been awake for a long period of time, sleep/wake homeostasis tells us that the need for sleep is increasing and that it is time to sleep. The biological clock and homeostatic drive act together so that we are alert during the day and asleep at night.

So What is the Solution?

Ask yourself the following questions:

1. Are you sleeping properly at night?
2. What are your sleeping habits?
3. Are you addicted to any gadgets?
4. Are you spending some time on yourself?

If the answer to most questions is 'no', then all you need to do is to follow a few important things listed below:

• After coming home from office, the first thing to do is to relax.

- For dinner, have light food with less carbohydrates.
- Avoid stimulants, like tea, coffee, colas, etc., during the last half of the shift.
- Avoid TV/computer/Internet surfing just before going to bed.
- Before going to sleep, read books or listen to light music.
- Establish a relaxing bedtime routine.
- Make the room comfortable for sleep—temperature, sound and light should be controlled.

POOR SLEEP DUE TO A RACING MIND
Case Study

There was the case of a twenty-five-year-old man—an engineer. He had been suffering from disturbed sleep (fragmented sleep) for four years, since his college days. Initially, he had this problem for about one year after which it improved, but then it recurred. For the last three years, his sleep had been very disturbed, he had trouble falling asleep (delayed onset), with occasional fragmentation of sleep. During sleep, he tended to think a lot and had vivid dreams. Naturally, the day was bad—he felt tired even when he'd just woken up, with fatigue only increasing during the day. Naturally, he was having trouble concentrating on his work.

Let's take a look at his day and night schedule. His bedtime is 10.30 or 11 p.m. The sleep onset is around

12–1 a.m. He wakes up at 3–4 a.m., has difficulty going back to sleep and is out of bed at around 7 a.m. He then heads out to work at 9 a.m., is back from office by 6.30 p.m. or 7 p.m., rests for a while, cooks his dinner, and then tries to plan for bedtime and how to get good sleep.

He is a non-smoker and doesn't drink alcohol; his tea intake is two or three cups a day; he does not consumer coffee and cola. His physical activity is nil. Luckily for him, his weight has remained stable. He's been told that he snores occasionally, more so when in a supine position (there is increased snoring in the supine position as the airway closure is maximum, with the collapse of tongue and palate).

He had been prescribed mood elevators (these increase the level of serotonin, the feel-good hormone in the body), Selective Serotonin Reuptake Inhibitors (SSRIs), hypnotics (sleep inducing pills), and anti-anxiety medication, which he was apprehensive to consume as he was worried about the side effects, dependence, etc.

So What is the Solution?

The ideal solution is to follow strict principles of sleep hygiene. These are a set of general rules and have to be dealt with one by one, especially those that are particularly relevant to the individual seeking a solution.

In this particular case, here are the important things I suggested the patient should focus on:

- Decrease discussion on sleep and not think of sleep all day.

- Reduce his intake of tea to one or two cups daily, and not after 5 p.m.
- Start with physical activity (such as a brisk walk) for thirty–forty minutes daily.
- Switch off all gadgets at least thirty minutes before going to sleep.
- Not keep lying in bed waiting for sleep. If unable to fall asleep in thirty minutes, he should get out of bed and read or listen to light music.

To allay his anxiety about snoring, and to assess his quality of sleep, I also got an overnight sleep test done, which revealed decreased sleep efficiency with mild snoring, but no other abnormality. After two months of following the routine suggested to him, his ability to sleep improved, with a decrease in 'awakenings' at night, and he woke up less tired. As a result, his days also improved. He made more friends at a sports club and became a happier person. In fact, I saw him smiling away on his follow-up visit.

He told me frankly, 'This is a heavenly feeling . . . I almost forgot what good sleep feels like.'

PARASOMNIA

Case Study

M. Singh, a seventeen-year-old student residing in Delhi, was diagnosed with parasomnia—a disorder characterized by abnormal or unusual behaviour of the nervous system during sleep. He used to walk in his sleep. He usually went to sleep by 11 p.m. and woke up at 6 a.m. In a month, he would feel fatigued more than once. Fortunately, he never fell asleep during daytime or while driving a vehicle and did not have high blood pressure. He developed this habit of sleepwalking in his childhood and he used to sleepwalk in the first half of the night. He usually slept with his mother or sister and it took him thirty–forty minutes to enter a sleep wave.

After some time, the parasomnia would start, and he would sit up and point at the wall and say things (called 'sleep talking' in sleep terminology). He talked in his sleep quite frequently. He could be easily put back to sleep and he had no memory of this unusual behaviour when he woke up. The only accident which could be traced in the patient's history was when he tripped while sleepwalking and ended up cutting his lower lip. He usually woke up at 6 a.m. and went to college by 7:30 a.m., and then play video games for five–six hours and used to watch TV before sleeping. Nothing 'wrong' really could be detected in his daily routine which could have been a cause for his behaviour. The only thing was that he used to study till late in the night when he was in class XII.

So What is the Solution?

This boy suffered from a combination of sleepwalking and sleep talking. These can co-exist or occur separately. The usual causes are poor sleep hygiene or if the parents or siblings suffer from a similar problem.

It can, however, cause a lot of worry, and can often result in injuries.

For him, I suggested he avoid gaming late at night, and start or incorporate some relaxing habits closer to bedtime. These simple changes have helped, and the episodes have reduced and are much milder.

GROANING IN SLEEP

A sixty-eight-year-old lady from Jaipur came to meet me with her son. She complained that she had been producing a loud sound in her sleep for over twenty years. Initially, this was mild and lower in volume, but over time it had become very loud, regular, and could even be heard outside the door and on the street. This resulted in considerable embarrassment to her and her family. She had been seen, investigated and evaluated by numerous lung specialists and neurologists.

The son had recorded a video of her, which was of great help.

I conducted an overnight sleep test with video recording to understand her condition further. It was important to know at what stage of sleep this occured, and also assess her breathing, snoring, etc. We discovered that the groaning occurred in her NREM sleep, soon after she fell asleep, and was very loud.

A device called positive airway pressure (PAP), which keeps the airway open, was used to blow air via a mask on her face, and that helped decrease the sound. She was told to use this regularly. PAP is the most common treatment for OSA.

It results in:

- Elimination of snoring and abnormal breathing events.
- Reduces daytime sleepiness.
- Improves blood pressure and blood sugar levels.
- Improves quality of life.

Tips to Adjust to PAP Therapy

➢ Use the right machine (CPAP/ BIPAP, fixed/auto, whatever is suggested) at the pressures suggested by the treating sleep expert.

➢ Use your machine (CPAP/BIPAP/AVAP) every night, making it a part of your bedtime routine.

➢ Use the nasal/full face mask/nasal pillow/headgear of the right fit so as to have the best level of comfort.

➢ If the sound of the machine is too loud/annoying, place a mouse pad under the machine to reduce the sound.

➢ If you feel the pressure is too high, use the 'ramp' mode; it will gradually increase the pressure, allowing you to fall asleep before increasing pressure to the desired level.

➢ If you have dryness in mouth/throat/nose, use a humidifier that fits well with your machine.

➢ If you experience nasal congestion, use a mild spray. If the problem is severe, try a nasal decongestant.

➢ Regular follow up with the sleep doctor is a must to make sure that you are using the machine/mask correctly and at the right pressures.

Care of Your CPAP

This will improve the effectiveness and also prolong the life of the equipment.

Daily Cleaning and Maintenance

Disconnect the air tubing and hang it in a clean, dry place. Hand-wash the mask with a mild detergent (e.g. Genteel) and leave to dry.

Weekly Cleaning and Maintenance

- Wash the mask and tubing with a mild detergent, rinse with water and hang to dry.
- Clean the device with a damp cloth.
- Inspect the mask, air tubing for wear-and-tear.
- Check the air filter for blockages due to dust, etc.

Do Not

- Use bleach, alcohol or spirit to clean the parts of the machine.
- Wash or dry the parts at high temperature or direct sunlight.
- Attempt to open and repair the CPAP.

Replacement

- Air Filter: Usually every three months or earlier, if it is a very dusty environment
- Mask: Every year
- Air Tubing: Every year

Humidifier

- Clean the humidifier tub with warm water and mild detergent, and wipe it dry.
- Change its water on a daily basis and add filtered/RO/soft water to it.
- Don't fill water beyond the maximum level.

BRUXISM/GRINDING OF TEETH

A thirty-two-year-old lady walked into my clinic one day, with her husband. She suffered from severe jaw pain. At night, she would wake up and find herself grinding her teeth. Her husband, too, was very disturbed by not only the noise but also by observing his wife and seeing how distressed she was. The patient admitted to feeling very low, and having bouts of sadness and poor sleep.

She had been advised to wear a night guard (which is worn over the teeth while sleeping, to prevent the teeth from rubbing against each other—something like what boxers wear), but the grinding still persisted.

Bruxism or teeth grinding can occur due to many reasons:

- Sleepwalking
- REM sleep disorders
- Anxiety or depression
- Sleep apnoea
- Nail biting
- Snoring
- Dementia

- Parkinsonism
- Stress (this being the most common factor)

I asked the patient to meet a psychologist and concluded that there was increased anxiety. So I advised her relaxation exercises, such as Jacobson's relaxation technique, pranayama, chanting of 'Om', and also prescribed a mild anti-anxiety medication. Overall, these measures greatly helped her and she improved in a few months.

SLEEP PARALYSIS

A twenty-two-year-old engineering student from IIT-Delhi came to the clinic looking very scared. He had been having episodes in his sleep where he couldn't move. He had a sense of impending doom, and an immense fear that someone was sitting on his chest and squeezing the air out of him.

This had been happening for the past six months. He was absolutely fine during the day. He denied any drug or substance abuse.

This is a typical episode of sleep paralysis; it usually occurs in highly stressed individuals. It is an intrusion of REM sleep into wakefulness, thus the individual is awake but feels paralysed. These episodes are self-limiting and usually last only for a few seconds.

I reassured him and explained the cause, and that this would not result in complete and permanent paralysis. This helped him understand the symptoms and he left feeling better. I did add that he should stop studying at a given time and then do something light before going to sleep, like listening to light music or reading a book.

He came back after three months and said he was feeling a lot better.

SEXSOMNIA

A nineteen-year-old boy came to my clinic, accompanied by his father. He requested his father to wait outside and then, after securing all the doors, he made me promise that I would not talk about the issue he was about to discuss with me to his father.

He was thoroughly embarrassed as his girlfriend complained to him one morning that she received very profane text messages from him after midnight. She was horrified because he spoke in a language he usually never used.

He was extremely surprised to see the messages, not just because of the content but also because had no recollection of writing those messages. He passed it off as a one-time occurrence.

However, the next episode was more horrifying. He attempted to fondle his sister while sleeping next to her. She woke up and shook him awake. He couldn't face her or himself, and was extremely ashamed and mortified.

This episode shook him and he decided to meet a sleep specialist and understand his condition. Why was this happening to him? What could he do to stop it?

This is a condition called sexsomnia, i.e. involuntary sexual acts during sleep with no recollection of it the morning after. The trigger for this, too, is sleep deprivation, as for all other parasomnias.

The patient had been partying extensively, sleeping at 4 a.m., and staying awake sometimes beyond that, and had also been smoking and drinking.

I simply suggested that he sleep and wake up on time, avoid alcohol and smoking, and these episodes would definitely die down; sure enough they did. He visited me after many months, fully cured.

In conclusion, as a sleep specialist, my message for everyone is: don't ignore sleep problems, no matter how minor. Seek medical advice and solutions at the earliest to prevent a minor problem from becoming a major sleep problem that can affect your creativity and your entire life. Solutions to your sleep problems are bound to improve the overall quality of your life.

Key Points for Better Sleep

- Sleep timing is a vital factor, besides sleep duration and quality.
- Decrease in sleep duration can produce severe disturbance such as parasomnias, sleep talking, sleepwalking with harm caused to one self and others.
- Ensure your sleep duration and timing is fixed to prevent the occurrence of parasomnias.

- It is crucial to relax the brain prior to sleep to avoid sleep disturbances.

SLEEPWALKING

Sleep disorders are of various kinds, such as sleepwalking, sleep talking, violent behaviour while asleep, lack of sleep and so on. Obviously, diagnosing and treating them correctly is of utmost importance. And just as obviously, questions are often asked about sleep disorders and their treatment.

For example, is sleepwalking in a child a source of concern? Here again, is an illustrative case study. A distraught, extremely anxious mother walked into my clinic one day with her beautiful, young daughter. I was amazed—what could be wrong with this adorable seven-year-old child? The mother narrated a story that left me speechless.

The night before they visited me, the mother woke up and went to the kitchen to get some water. To her horror, she saw someone standing in the balcony of her eighth-floor apartment. Her initial reaction was that it was an intruder, but she quickly realized that the person was a child. She discovered that it was her own daughter, looking around, apparently very confused.

'No words can describe what I went through for those few moments,' the mother said. 'I walked slowly towards her, and then snatched her up in my arms and rushed inside.' The mother barely slept for the rest of the night. She rushed to my clinic in the morning, terrified to think about what could have happened and that it might happen again.

To identify the cause fully, I had to understand the child's day and night routine. What time did she sleep? What did she do last before falling asleep? Did she watch scary TV shows, etc.? Here are the answers provided by her mother:

- She slept in her own room.
- Parents often think that children fall asleep after saying good night. However, most do not. In this case, the child used to watch shows on TV and then read till 11 p.m. She had to wake up for school at 6 a.m., at which point in time she felt very tired and lethargic.
- The mother also mentioned that her husband used to sleepwalk as a child, but then outgrew the habit.

After getting this information, I worked out the night-time and day activities for the child and her mother. I discussed the importance of getting adequate sleep, doing a relaxing activity prior to sleep, and specially avoiding TV at night.

It was clearly a case of sleepwalking, which is known to occur in children, before it gradually subsides. Children usually outgrow it by nine–ten years of age. Sleepwalking can occur when wakefulness intrudes into sleep. To ensure this doesn't recur, the following things should be done:

- Establish a good bedtime routine.
- Ensure adequate duration of sleep—an eight-year-old ideally requires nine hours of sleep.
- Keep a fixed bedtime and waking up time.

- Don't allow a child to use gadgets, watch TV, etc., before going to sleep. Switch them off at least an hour before turning the lights off.

The mother met me a month later, looking much happier and shared her daughter's routine with me. She was getting eight–nine hours of sleep at night and appeared more rested, was waking up for school easily, with no further episodes of sleepwalking.

Sleepwalking Causing Serious Injury

I once had a twenty-four-year-old, extremely bright boy come to my clinic with his worried, distressed parents. He had recently graduated from an engineering programme in the US and was working there. The parents lived in India.

The story they shared was a blood-curdling one— he was found walking at night on the streets in the freezing cold, with blood dripping down his right leg, and a fixed stare on his face. Fortunately, he was rushed to a nearby hospital where they detected a torn artery in his leg and immediately operated upon him, thus saving his life.

This boy had a history of sleepwalking in the past, although only occasionally. On questioning him, the following details emerged: he had a certain project which he had to complete soon, thus he barely slept for three– four hours at night. On the night of the event, he slept at 4 a.m. and, apparently during the sleepwalking episode, walked out through the open double glass windows, injuring an artery in the leg, and continued to walk down the street, in the snow, oblivious to his wound.

Obviously, the parents were extremely distressed and were not sure if they could send him back to the US. He was to get married in a few months.

After much discussion and counselling during the sessions, I explained sleep need, duration, sleep debt and hazards of inadequate sleep to him. Finally, he understood the necessity of sleeping on time and keeping regular sleep/wake schedules.

The parents visited me after a few months with the wedding invite and with the good news that the patient was doing well, with no further sleepwalking episodes.

Anyone facing such a problem should maintain strict sleep hygiene principles, and fix a bedtime and wake-up time.

RESTLESS LEGS SYNDROME

People with Restless Legs Syndrome (RLS) face difficulty in falling asleep because they suffer discomfort or pain, with the urge to move their legs at bedtime, which gets relieved on the movement. In our country, other measures such as massaging, pressing, tying a cloth also work for some. Such people may also experience similar complaints during long flights or while sitting in a car for long periods of time with or without the jerking of legs during sleep.

RLS can be caused by certain medical conditions and also medication:

- Low blood iron levels
- Diabetes
- Pregnancy
- Kidney disorders
- Certain vitamins or mineral deficiencies
- Nerve problems in the spine or legs
- Poor blood circulation in the legs
- Genetic
- Antidepressants and anti-nausea medicines worsen RLS

The symptoms cause difficulty in falling asleep and result in poor quality of sleep, which leads to tiredness during the day. RLS symptoms may interfere with the ability to sit for long meetings, watch movies, or car and plane rides.

Most people suffering from RLS have jerking movements of legs in sleep, resulting in 'brief awakenings'. These can lead to increased blood pressure, blood sugar levels, etc.

Treatment of RLS

RLS can be improved by changes in behaviour, and/or treated with medication.

Behavioural Changes

- Regular exercise
- Massaging the legs when symptoms occur

- Mental exercise such as calculations at bedtime
- Decrease coffee/tea/caffeine intake
- Stop smoking
- Reducing stress
- Avoid alcohol

Some home-based remedies

- Hot baths
- Heat application
- Ice packs

There are many medicines available to treat RLS. However, these should only be consumed when recommended by a specialist.

Violent Behaviour and Self-Injury During Sleep

Among the many interesting cases that have come to me, there were several which involved violent behaviour and self injury during sleep. There was, for example, a docile, meek person who was a thorough gentleman during the day, but a completely changed person at night—violent, aggressive, abusive. It was almost unbelievable that it was the same person, somewhat like Dr Jekyll and Mr Hyde.

A sixty-three-year-old gentleman visited me with episodes of abnormal behaviour during his sleep. Sometimes, he woke up with a big bruise as he had hit his leg on the wall at night. Once he even fell off the bed and hurt his head. When asked how and why it happened, all that he could remember was he had a very bad dream in which someone was attacking him and he was trying to protect himself.

The family tried their own preventive measures like placing a mattress next to his bed. However, he developed new forms of violence. He started shouting at night, talking very loudly at times, and occasionally emitting blood-curdling screams. This sometimes continued for hours, resulting in the entire family suffering, in addition to causing extreme worry about his condition. His days were normal as usual and he had no recollection of his nightly behaviour, in which he was a different personality altogether. Naturally, the family was very concerned and had questions: What was his condition? Why did it occur and how could it be stopped?

As explained earlier, we have two stages of sleep—NREM and REM. There is an inherent protective mechanism during REM sleep: the brain is very active but the body remains motionless. This is a natural and important protective mechanism. Can you imagine what would happen if we moved, talked, etc., in our dreams? However, if the brain areas which control REM sleep are damaged or are involved abnormally, the protective mechanism can break down, leading to a condition or disorder called dream enactment, which is what had happened in the case of this patient.

Fortunately, this disorder can be controlled, which we did by prescribing a single tablet at night for the patient. It worked like magic for him and his entire family. Gradually, the screaming stopped and everyone in the family was able to enjoy the power of restorative sleep once again. Obviously, it is worth re-emphasizing the importance of sleep, and the havoc that lack of sleep can wreak in an individual's life and often in the lives of the individual's family members as well.

Key Points for Better Sleep

- Sleep disorders are of various kinds such as sleepwalking, sleep talking, violent behaviour while sleeping, lack of sleep and so on. Fortunately, they can all be treated by a sleep specialist.
- Sleepwalking is known to occur in children. They usually outgrow it by nine–ten years of age.
- To ensure this doesn't keep recurring, establish a good bedtime routine and ensure adequate duration of sleep—an eight-year-old ideally requires nine hours of sleep.
- Keep a fixed bedtime and waking up time.
- Don't allow a child to use gadgets, watch TV, etc., prior to sleep. Switch them off at least an hour before turning the lights off.

11

SLEEP AND TECHNOLOGY

These days, a lot of patients walk in to my clinic with data collected from 'apps for sleep'. There are numerous types of applications that either record sleep, induce sleep or help you wake up from sleep. There is, for example, the sleep cycle alarm clock adjusted to wake you up at your lightest sleep time with soothing tunes (to avoid waking you up from slow wave sleep, which can leave you feeling very groggy).

There are various apps available on Android and iOS platforms which help you get sound sleep. The apps available are:

- Sleep—soothing sound, lullabies
- Deep sleep—guided meditation
- Insomnia cure
- Yoga for insomnia
- Relax and sleep
- Sleepmaker rain
- Nature sounds
- Sleep soundly hypnosis—'guided relaxation session'

HOW EFFECTIVE ARE GADGETS AND DEVICES?

A major query arises: do these apps, gadgets and devices like an iPad, etc., really help one get good sleep? My answer as a sleep specialist is: I'm not sure. They're probably good for a brief period of time, but anything that keeps you constantly thinking about sleep and worrying about it, will make sleep more difficult to get. The harder you try, the more it will evade you.

Yet, many people turn to gadgets to help them sleep. They might be fun to use, but they are no substitute for good sleeping habits, like going to bed at the same time every night, minimizing caffeine and relaxing before bedtime. 'Gadgets can be helpful, but their effectiveness does not supersede sleep awareness and good sleep and circadian hygiene,' says Gianluca Tosini, MD, director of the Circadian Rhythm and Sleep Disorders Program at the Neuroscience Institute, and chairman of the department of pharmacology at Morehouse School of Medicine in Atlanta.[1]

The Perfect Night's Sleep Starts Long Before You Get Into Bed

Searching for the ever-elusive perfect night's sleep? Prevent sleep sabotage by sticking to this pre-bedtime timeline.

HOURS BEFORE BED ▶

| 6 HRS | 5 HRS | 4 HRS | 3 HRS | 2 HRS | 1 HR | BED |

Stop drinking caffeine

Stop drinking alcohol

Finish exercising

Turn off electronics

Night, night!

Finish eating dinner (2–3 hours)

Stop working, studying & stressing

Sources: National Sleep Foundation, Michael A. Grandner, Ph.D., WebMD

THE HUFFINGTON POST

Good Habits and Sleep

Here are some easy-to-adopt, very beneficial good habits for inducing sleep:

• Unwind early

I know many people who set a deadline to sleep by 10 p.m. but struggle to finish off the day's chores until 9.59 p.m.! Plan ahead so it doesn't feel like a race against time. You should ideally switch off your television set forty–sixty minutes before you go to bed.

• Avoid big meals at night

Attending a late-night party? Avoid oil-laden foods and big meals at night as they might bother you later.

• Limit your alcohol intake

I know a non-drinker who would consume a glass of white wine on flights just so it could help him fall asleep faster. Consuming alcohol in moderation is fine, but don't go overboard as too much alcohol reduces the quality of sleep and one is likely to wake up early morning with a dry mouth and a headache.

• Limit intake of caffeine

Some people can have sleep problems from caffeine consumed ten hours ago! Why not switch to water or herbal tea after lunch?

- Relax with a bedtime ritual

Establish a bedtime routine that stimulates relaxation. This could be anything—like taking a hot bath, doing slow stretches, listening to soft music, deep breathing or sipping on a warm cup of chamomile tea. Dim the lights, as that is believed to induce the production of melatonin, the hormone that helps one fall, and stay, asleep.

- Set a sleep schedule

Fix a time by when you wish to go off to sleep and stick to it as best as you can. By doing this, your body will get into a routine and ensure you have a good night's rest.

- Refrain from napping during the day

I advise patients to refrain from daytime napping unless it is absolutely essential. A long daytime nap can lead to trouble sleeping at night. If you really want to catch a nap in the daytime, make it thirty minutes or less.

- Use aromatherapy

Essential oils like rose, chamomile, juniper, lavender and sandalwood all have a sedative effect when inhaled. Rub a wee bit on the insides of your wrists or on your temples and breathe in the relaxing fragrance as you drift into dreamland.

I would like to share a story with you. Her friends called her Gadget Ganapati. She was fifteen years old, and was always occupied with her phone or iPad. She is the daughter of a diplomat and has travelled extensively with her father. She has friends all over the world, in different time zones. One fine day, her mother visited me. She was greatly concerned about her daughter's sleep timings and duration, mood changes and increased appetite at night, with a 10 kg weight gain.

She usually went to sleep at 3–4 a.m. in the morning, and, with great difficulty, would wake up at 7 a.m. for school. Throughout the night, she chatted with her friends from different countries. It was no surprise then that she couldn't wake up for school, was groggy and irritable on being woken up, with increasing absenteeism. To fight this sleep drive, she discovered an energy drink. She started with gulping a can of the drink daily, which increased to three–four cans a day. She snapped continuously, was very irritable, moody, and lost her cool easily. As she stayed awake late at night, she tended to munch on snacks, whatever she could find, leading to an increase in weight. It soon became a difficult situation to handle.

Solution

To help her, I had to understand what her problem was, and how I could get her to help herself. Was she concerned about her weight, mood swings and performance? Only by getting her on board and having her co-operate could I help her. I explained the logic behind weight gain and poor sleep, the role of sleep in maintaining one's mood, and scholastic performance to her. She understood and decided to help herself mend her habits. Within a few weeks, she was a pleasant, happy child with increased school attendance and performance.

Incidentally, gadgets have not only affected the youth and children but have also affected the elderly. To my surprise, an elegant, well-groomed seventy-eight-year-old lady came to visit me with the problem of fragmented sleep. She was able to fall asleep between 11 p.m.–12 a.m. The onset of sleep was very good, but around 2–3 a.m., she would wake up and find it difficult to fall asleep. At this point, she would surf the Internet, update her Facebook, etc., using her iPad. As time passed, she would play games and read, etc., and on a few days, would see the sun rise and then realize that the night was over. She would feel a bit sleepy around 6 a.m., and would take a nap for an hour, until 7 a.m., after which she would get out of bed and have a miserable day, with a heavy head and puffy eyes. By the afternoon, the fatigue would increase and she would take a nap for one–two hours, post lunch. This became her routine, and she was very disturbed as the night became a thing to be afraid of. 'Will I ever be able to sleep continuously?' was her constant fear.

We do know that there is a tendency for some people to wake up in the middle of the night. In fact, Dr Klaus Ekrich has done extensive research on this and called it 'Ekrich's Theory of Non-consolidated Sleep'. This was a common occurrence among our ancestors and only with industrialization has it become continuous, consolidated sleep. Another important point to consider is that the elderly have fragmented sleep, poor quality of sleep with decrease in slow wave sleep, resulting in 'awakenings' at night. Thus, the causes of sleep fragmentation in this particular patient's case were numerous, and we had to help her accordingly.

Solution

The first thing was to discuss the effects of aging on sleep with her and explain a few facts about sleep in the elderly. This is called cognitive training. Further, we needed to make her understand the effect of the light from an iPad on sleep. An iPad emits a blue light of the wavelength 450–495 nm, which suppresses the melatonin, resulting in wakefulness. This resulted in her inability to go back to sleep. Her naps were further responsible for her sleep fragmentation. The build of sleep drive is essential during the day (homeostatic drive for control of sleep), and is responsible for maintaining sleep. Frequent naps disturb this drive and cause poor quality of sleep. She was advised to rest for thirty minutes in the afternoon and not longer.

To the patient's surprise, these seemingly simple suggestions caused a remarkable change in her sleep pattern, which gradually developed into a habit. In case she did wake up, she was advised not to worry or panic, not to pick up the iPad, and was gradually able to fall asleep again. This goes to prove that sleep hygiene tips work wonders. (see Chapter 16 on Sleep Hygiene).

Hopefully, I have been able to convince you of the adverse effects of technology/devices on our sleep. It's not that one should avoid being tech savvy. However, when to use it, and how much time to use it for are important things to remember. According to some, surfing for information about sleep on the Internet can provide self-help techniques to achieve uninterrupted sleep. But to be able to filter information correctly, one must learn what to avoid and what to do. Some devices can actually help, or at least trigger, a sleep-inducing effect.

Key Points for Better Sleep

- It is good to be tech savvy, but when and how much to use these gadgets are things to be considered. And this should definitely not be the last thing one does before going to bed.
- Frequent naps during the day disturb the sleep drive and cause poor quality of sleep.
- Follow simple tips to induce sleep; one must learn what to avoid and what to do.
- Some devices can help, or at least trigger, a sleep-inducing effect.

12

THE ADVERSE EFFECTS OF TECHNOLOGY

Does technology have an adverse impact on sleep? In this technology-driven age of gizmos and gadgets, should one consider technology a bane or a boon in terms of tackling sleep and sleep-related problems? Both these questions are debatable. I will discuss a few cases where the use of technology in day-to-day life has actually had an adverse impact on sleep patterns.

Mr R was a thirty-two-year-old bright, good looking young man, working as a consultant with an international company. He was happily married and had two children. The desire to become successful is what drives many people these days and before they realize it, that's all their life becomes—a struggle for success, at the cost of many other vital things in life. That's what happened in the case of Mr R too, who soon realized that in this competitive race, he had become a loner and, therefore, was soon completely cut off from his family.

How and why did this happen? Every waking moment of the day, he was on his smartphone or iPad, constantly working. This became such an integral part of his life that even while having a conversation with his wife or children, he was found looking at a screen instead of the person's eyes. This gradually led to his exclusion from family matters.

'In fact I didn't even realize when my wife moved into a separate bedroom. It happened so gradually, and I guess I was totally lost in my world,' he said.

'However, I guess this had to have an effect on me sometime—I soon discovered I couldn't fall asleep, and once I slept I woke up very frequently. This resulted in extreme exhaustion on waking up, with difficulty in performing my tasks at work and mood swings where I found myself snapping at people. From a pleasant, happy person, I realized I had transformed into a very irritable one. How and when did this happen, and why? These questions arose and I felt I should do something about this, so I discovered an app which records one's sleep and also suggests ways to improve it, the best time to wake up, etc. I followed this diligently for a month, but to my horror the situation only seemed to be getting worse. Then I went back to refer to the Internet, and to my surprise found that there were specialists who can help with this and discovered Dr Bhatia on Google. She spent about an hour with me, understood my daily routine, my work, family relationships, any medication, habits (smoking, consumption of alcohol) hobbies, etc. I detailed my twenty-four-hour day and night routine for her.

- Wake up by 7 a.m., reach office at 9 a.m.
- The day is very hectic, continuous meetings, brain-storming sessions with frequent cups of coffee.

- Finally finish by 8 p.m.
- Home by 8.30 p.m.
- Head to the gym—9 p.m. to 9:30 p.m., for a workout.
- Dinner by 10:30 p.m.
- Check some more emails, watch the news for a short time.
- Sleeping time: 11:30 p.m. Since I find it difficult to fall asleep, I start surfing the Internet my phone; time flies and it's around 1 a.m.
- I turn on the sleep application on the mobile to track my sleep.

'After an in-depth discussion, I was recommended a few basic things/tips. It was a surprise to me that I had come to meet a specialist and I was being told things that are very basic. So I left the clinic with a lot of reservation and doubts about how these things would work out for me and improve my sleep.'

According to Mr R, the application was helping him to understand his sleep and sleep better. He came with a month's data on the application. After assessing his routine, it was apparent that Mr R was consuming too much of coffee during the day and sometimes till late in the evening, which blocks the receptors. A receptor is a protein molecule usually found fixed within the plasma membrane surface of a cell that receives chemical signals from outside. In simpler terms, the receptors act like an on–off switch for a particular activity in the cell. If the right substance comes along that fits into the receptor—like a key fitting into a lock—the switch is turned on and a particular activity in the cell begins.

This application is easily available in the mobile playstore. The application demonstrates how to keep a track of sleep, and even provides a lullaby if one has problems in sleeping.

The images below will explain this process stepwise:

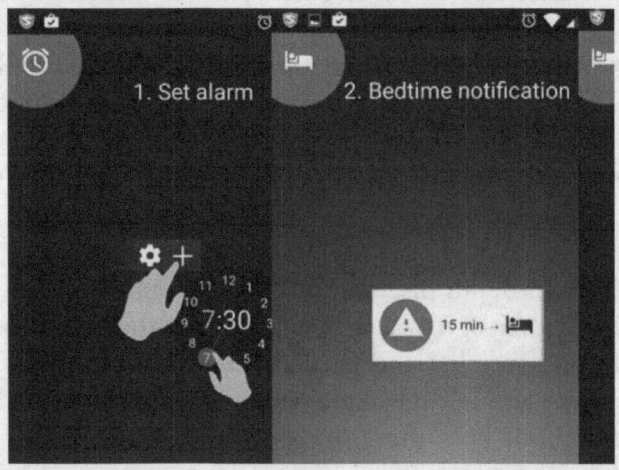

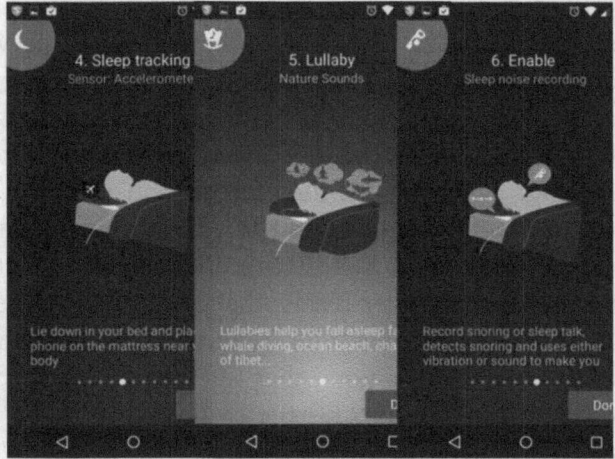

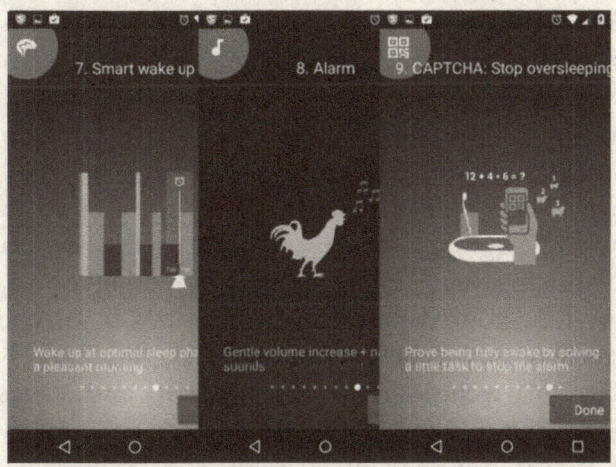

I suggested decreasing stimulation—whether in food or exercise. Caffeine blocks the adenosine receptors, which are responsible for inducing sleep. Thus, coffee produces wakefulness. I pinpointed that apart from caffeine, in Mr R's case, his late visits to the gym were also affecting his sleep cycle. Exercise acts like a stimulant, causing excessive sympathetic stimulation, thus interfering with the onset of sleep.

The tendency to spend the last few hours of the day, prior to sleep, on gadgets was resulting in a further delay in sleep by suppressing the release of melatonin.

Most importantly, he had no 'me time'. In every individual's life, 'me time' is very important, as it is very commonly said, one must not forget oneself in the race to be first. In Mr R's case, he was constantly on the move the whole day—there was no time for hobbies, none to just sit, relax, laugh, etc., which are necessary in one's daily schedule.

Some quality time spent with one's own self helps keep the mind in a peaceful state. This peace of mind helps us relax and wind down. It is even suggested to set a 'worry time' early in the evening, so as to clear the mind of any stress of jobs that need to be done.

One doesn't need to be a sleep specialist to figure out where Mr R was going wrong. In fact, many people lead similar lives. The technique of noting down the twenty-four-hour day and night activities is, of course, an excellent tool to help a person realize this.

I got a psychologist to assess Mr R, and it was no surprise that he had a typical type A personality—a kind of person who wants everything to be perfect, and lead a perfect life.

Some questions I asked him were:

- Have you recently gone on a vacation?
- What are you hobbies?

In Mr R's case, it was essential to take some time off immediately.

Here is a list of things I suggested specifically to help improve his sleep. They are applicable to everybody and especially for those in the same age group as Mr R.

- Avoid using the application to track sleep; it will cause more anxiety.
- Stop worrying about sleep.
- Take out some time for relaxation.
- Decrease coffee intake; avoid coffee altogether after 12 noon.
- Visits to the gym should always be before 7 p.m.
- Establish a relaxing pre-bedtime routine.

- Play with the children; read to them.
- Switch off all gadgets an hour before lights off.

Are you curious to know what all this resulted in? In the patient's own words, 'Doctor, thank you for showing me that life has much more to offer, and I also want to thank you for re-introducing me to my children. I enjoy my time with them, sleep peacefully and my colleagues are also happy with me.'

After following a month-long rigorous routine, Mr R and his wife are once again together in the bedroom, and now Mr R spends quality time in the morning and evening with his children. He drops them to school and plays with them in the evening. On the whole, he is a much happier, much more amicable person. According to him, simple tips and rules can work wonders if we're willing to give them a try. If you really want to lead a good life (personal and professional), all you need is some quality time for yourself.

Key Points for Better Sleep

- Exercising late in the evening or late visits to the gym can affect sleep. Exercise acts like a stimulant, causing excessive sympathetic stimulation, thus interfering with sleep onset.
- Decrease coffee intake; avoid it after 12 noon.
- The tendency to spend the last few hours prior to sleep on gadgets results in further delay in sleep by suppressing the release of melatonin.
- 'Me time' is required for good sleep. In every individual's life, 'me time' is very important. Simple tips and rules can work wonders if we're willing to give them a try.

13

SLEEP, LIFESTYLES AND SUBSTANCE ABUSE

It is important to understand how our behaviour, lifestyle and other factors play a major role in changing our sleep pattern. In my day-to-day practice, over the years, a very common problem I have observed among youngsters in particular is encapsulated in the words, 'Oh, I can't sleep!' I've dealt with this in an earlier chapter. In addition to this, sleep problems often have a relationship with substance abuse. Recently, for example, a twenty-three-year-old handsome, but extremely worried, young man, hailing from Jammu, walked in to see me. His problem, which came as no surprise, was, 'I can't sleep.'

As discussed in earlier chapters, this is actually a symptom. It is the cause behind 'I can't sleep' that needs to be determined. The question of 'Why?' needs to be answered. Only then can the solution be provided.

In the case of the young man from Jammu, he had recently moved to Delhi to attend coaching classes in order to appear for entrance exams. Back home in Jammu, there had always been a desire to stay awake all night, but parental supervision didn't allow that to happen.

In Delhi, however, away from his parents, with no one to regulate his 'sleep–wake' cycle, there was total freedom. So he stayed awake through the nights, surfing the Internet or watching movies, and slept intermittently during the day. This pattern continued for two–three months. The repercussions followed soon enough. He was not able to wake up for the morning classes, absenteeism increased, which led to him falling behind in projects. He realized that he should sleep by 11 p.m. to wake up at 6 a.m. So he tried going to sleep at 11 p.m., but to his horror and surprise, he just couldn't. Some of his 'wise' friends suggested he should try alcohol to help him fall asleep. After a while, he yielded to the idea, which worked initially, but then led to an increase in the quantity of alcohol being consumed. Soon enough, smoking and imbibing other addictive substances followed. What was the status of sleep in all this? Some nights were good and some bad; some days were good and some bad.

Coaching classes had become secondary, and all the goals in his life had shifted. Fortunately, good sense prevailed soon and the veil lifted from his eyes. He realized this was not what he had left his home for, but when he tried to stop and change it, his sleep deteriorated further and so did his mood and concentration. That's what induced him to seek help. The good thing was his motivation to come out of all this, and, of course, his need to get some good sleep.

After an extensive session with him, and one with a counsellor, I was able to make him understand the role of the body clock, how he had tampered with it, re-set it, resulting in his inability to fall asleep. The alcohol and other substances, I pointed out to him, do help initiate sleep but cause fragmentation of sleep and this was leaving him tired upon waking up.

I also stressed on the importance of physical activity—thirty to forty-five minutes daily—and the role of blue light in gadgets, which suppresses melatonin, thus interfering with sleep. My suggestion to him was that he should switch off all gadgets an hour before sleeping.

He was used to having a rich, oily dinner at 10 p.m. Here again, I suggested he change it to an early and light dinner. Heavy food at night is hard to digest and also disturbs sleep.

Further, I handed him a sheet—a sleep diary (refer to page 58 for more details)—to fill, so that he could appreciate how his day and night went.

As his motivation was very high, he did exactly as he was told, and when he returned with his sleep diary after two weeks, matters had improved considerably.

'Why Am I So Tried and Sleepy during the Day?'

This is a common question asked nowadays by young people. Let's try and understand this through a case study. I am confident that by the time you've finished reading this and other case studies detailed here, you will be able to help not only yourself but also your colleagues, friends, relatives and others. How? By identifying their problems, and, in some cases, you will even be able to provide solutions. In this particular case, a handsome, cheerful, bright, but slightly obese young man, a thirty-year-old, walked in with a petite, beautiful and charming young wife. They were greeted by the obvious question, 'What brings you here?' The two exchanged embarrassed glances, and then they blurted out simultaneously, 'snoring'.

This opened the tap and the details came pouring out. The young man snored very loudly while sleeping. Not only that, his snores even changed tones, pitch and frequency, and he was even prone to stop breathing suddenly. This would be followed by a loud snore. He would suddenly sit up, and then go back to sleep with the snoring starting all over again.

He would wake up feeling lousy and could get to office only after consuming two strong cups of coffee. But after just a few hours at work, he would feel as if a curtain was gradually covering his eyes and brain. He had difficulty concentrating, couldn't focus during meetings and needed a few more cups of coffee to keep him going. He would somehow manage to get through the day. Back home, he would find, to his horror and amazement, that he had dozed off while sitting on a chair, watching TV. He had to cancel all social events, movies, dinners with friends, etc., because he simply didn't have the energy or desire. To top it all, he had gained about 10–12 kg in six months. Could all this be due to depression, he wondered? He couldn't believe this could be happening to him. It was at this point that a friend, who had been helped by me, suggested that he and his wife meet me.

After they had finished giving me the details of the problem, the first thing I did was to assure them that it was a remediable, reversible condition known as obstructive sleep apnoea (OSA).

To find the most effective solution, the patient's sleep would need to be monitored for one night, in what is termed an overnight sleep study.

Fortunately, the couple agreed that this should be done as soon as possible. The overnight sleep study observed the loud snoring, and noted that the pauses (apnoeas) were in large numbers and for long durations. At the end of each pause, the sleep would break. This resulted in frequent interruptions in sleep.

These cause a sympathetic surge which is responsible for a rise in blood pressure and insulin levels, changes in immunity, alterations in appetite stimulating hormones (ghrelin) and satiety control hormones (leptin), with an increased desire to eat starchy, carbohydrate-rich food.

The pauses in breathing are accompanied by a drop in oxygen saturation, with decreased oxygen flow to the brain, which can cause memory problems in the future and changes in the lining of the arteries.

The pauses in breathing, with repeated arousals, are responsible for the tired, un-refreshed feeling on waking up, greater fatigue during the day with increased sleepiness and poor concentration.

The patient and his wife were relieved to hear that all this could be corrected, and were glad that instead of considering snoring as a sign of good health and sound sleep, as advised by many, they had come to seek help. They were keen to know why all this occurs and how to remedy it.

I explained to them that the passage for breathing is a muscular pipe, starting from the nose and extending to the lungs. This pipe is open during the day and decreases mildly at night. When narrowing occurs, the passage of air in the narrowed airway causes snoring. When the pipe decreases further in diameter, there is complete cessation of air flow, causing a pause in breathing.

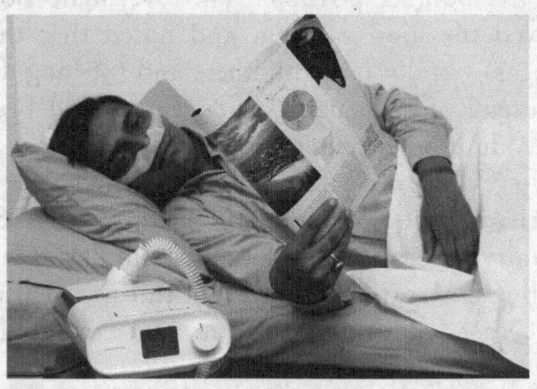

Fortunately, to correct all this, there is a device which can push air under pressure to open up the blocked airway and reverse all the changes that go with it. It looks like a box, weighs approximately 1 kg, and has a tube and a mask which fits on the face. The device takes in air from the outside and delivers it under pressure; this is usually determined by the night test, and varies for each person. The pressurized air stops the snoring, opens the airway and improves breathing. This results in improving the quality of sleep and improves the day too. The young man accepted my suggestion, worked on it, and after a week, the couple walked in to my clinic with smiles on their faces, exuberant that they were back in the same bedroom, and were enjoying spending time together in the evenings. He was back to being a cheerful, motivated and creative person at work.

The Curious Case of Sleeping Pills

Though many people with sleeping problems may share the same symptoms, each case has its own distinct elements. So far, the case studies shared with you have been from my view point. But in the case of RS, a housewife, it might be interesting to read in her own words the difficulties she experienced and how she found the solutions.

I was no older than forty-two when I lost my dearest son. That was twenty-five long years ago. Thereafter, I suffered from several problems, like unexplained extreme fatigue, feeling low, I had no desire to meet people and preferred to be alone. Along with it came difficulty in sleeping, and that's when I started taking sleeping pills. But soon, they stopped being effective and I had to increase the dose. However, to my horror, I found that in spite of increasing the dose, I would wake up four–five times at night, with difficulty in going back to sleep, with the result that I had to pull myself out of bed in the morning even as late as 8–9 a.m. It didn't end here. The whole day, I would look for an opportunity to take a nap, whether in the car, or while reading or watching TV and even during some family gathering. This became an embarrassing situation.

To add to this, I put on 20 kg, developed diabetes, which went totally out of control. The weight gain, the sleepless nights, horrible days and the sleeping pills became a part of my life.

One fine day, a friend of mine suggested going to a doctor named Manvir Bhatia. I went to her, accompanied by my husband, though I really didn't think anyone or anything could help me. I discussed my sleeping habits with her and then revealed that my sleep was very fragmented, with frequent trips to the washroom.

She listened to me very patiently and we discussed what could be going wrong. She then enquired if I snore—and my husband remarked: 'Yes, very loudly.'

She assured me that I would be able to go off the sleeping pills, but would have to be monitored for one night through a test called sleep study.

To my surprise, the results of the sleep study test were a total revelation. It confirmed very loud snoring, but also showed that I was having very long pauses in breathing—with a resultant drop in oxygen levels while sleeping. These pauses interrupted the sleep and a hormone released during this was the culprit which sent me to the washroom. Another important thing was that some other hormones that were being released were responsible for my craving for starchy, fried, sweet food and the resultant increase in my weight.

I was diagnosed to be suffering from sleep apnoea (a common disorder in which one has one or more pauses in breathing or shallow breathing while sleeping).

It was suggested I use a mask at night, which would deliver air under pressure, from a machine.

The idea was terrifying, and my first reaction was: 'Doctor, how can you expect me to wear such a mask and sleep?' Dr Bhatia made me understand the benefits of the mask. I was persuaded, and it was my good fortune that I agreed to try it. It worked as a boon in my life.

Since that day, there has been no looking back. My nights improved, my days improved, the diabetes is under control, and my weight has gradually started decreasing. The best part is I can breathe normally, and my son is happy to see me getting better. And here's something that happened way, way beyond my expectations— I've stopped taking sleeping pills.

As a doctor, I too am very pleased that RS was able to kick the pernicious habit of taking sleeping pills. One of the most dreadful things is dependence on sleeping pills— it's like an addiction; the body develops tolerance and demands an increase in the dose. It also causes a hangover-like effect during the day and deepens depression.

As the sampling of case studies in this shows, in each and every instance of sleep problems, simple solutions can work wonders—provided there is a desire to set things right. This requires no medication, only changes in lifestyle, but the challenge lies in making an individual understand why it should be done.

SK, a thirty-two-year-old engineer, came to me with the problem of insomnia. He was treated by some other doctor from 2009–2015, but he continued to have sleep issues and also felt very dull during the day, with mood swings, irritability, forgetfulness and decreased motivation in spite of taking medicines. He searched for sleep specialists and this led him to me.

'I visited her on 8 May 2015; she understood my problem, helped me to understand the role of sleep hygiene, and the harmful effects with continuous use of sleeping pills. She gave me alternate medication which was very good, gave me 80 per cent relief and was able to stop all the other multiple medicines that I was taking.

'On my next visit after three months, all medicines were stopped and I felt I had a new life. I shall be eternally grateful to her for helping me to stop the pills and improve my quality of life.'

What are Sleeping Pills?

Any drug that is used for the purpose of inducing or maintaining sleep is a sleeping pill. Sleeping pills are one of the most prescribed, as well as bought over-the-counter, pills used worldwide. There are various classes of sleeping pills, and they are classified into three major types—barbiturates, benzodiazepines and miscellaneous types—based on the chemical structure of molecules. Nevertheless, a vast majority of sleeping pills act by enhancing the amount or effect of gaba, a neurotransmitter that dampens nervous system impulses.

The most common sleeping pills prescribed in medical practice today come from the benzodiazepines. They include the commonly used brands of clonazepam, estazolam, etizolam, alprazolam and, rarely, diazepam.

They do cause a hangover-like effect the following day, and long-term use is associated with the development of tolerance, as a result of which a higher dose is required for the same sedating/hypnotic effect. Another major problem with benzodiazepines is dependence upon use for more than ten–fifteen days, and risk of rebound insomnia and withdrawal symptoms. The latter includes agitation, inattention, craving for pills, hypertension, tachycardia, etc.

A newer class of sleeping pills which we classify under the miscellaneous group includes the non-benzodiazepines hypnotics that include brands like zolpidem, zolpiclone, eszolpiclone, etc. Initially, they were marketed as drugs devoid of dependency potency, but these claims have been falsified to some extent.

Sleeping pills are lucrative options for anyone suffering from sleepless nights. Many people indulge in self-medication, but the harmful effects should be understood before using them.

Sleeping pills like clonazepam can cause drowsiness, poor concentration, ataxia (difficulty in walking), difficulty in speaking and driving, vision problems, muscle weakness, dizziness and mental confusion, and anterograde amnesia.

Considering these severe effects of using sleeping pills over short and long terms, it is essential to use them judiciously for the shortest term possible, with minimal dosage.

Key Points for Better Sleep

- Majority of sleep problems and conditions are remediable and reversible.
- Maintain a sleep diary for a while to appreciate how your day and night go.

- Simple solutions can work wonders, provided there is a desire to set things right. This requires no medication, only a change in lifestyle.
- Try and stick to an early, light dinner. Heavy food at night is hard to digest and also disturbs sleep.
- Switch off all gadgets an hour prior to sleep.
- There are remedies and devices available to help you bring problems like snoring and dependence on sleeping pills under control. But for this, you must seek guidance from an experienced and competent sleep doctor.

14

SLEEP AND RELATIONSHIPS

Does sleep affect relationships, especially when sharing a bedroom? Yes, sleep does affect relationships. In fact, as a sleep specialist, I was surprised to note how often it affects relationships and the various factors responsible for it. Let's discuss a few 'causative' points which I observed in my patients.

Various Factors Affecting Relationships

Different Sleep Timings

Consider this situation: It's bedtime for the wife at 9 p.m, and her wake up time is 4 a.m.—she has do to the morning puja as well as pack lunch for both her husband and her school-going children.

The husband's bedtime is midnight and wake up time is 8 a.m.

So what's the conflict? Obviously, both disturb each other's sleep due to the difference in timing.

Different Temperature Preferences

Women generally feel colder and prefer a warmer room temperature as compared to men, who prefer the room to be cooler. Yes, there is a scientific explanation for this.

Women have a higher body fat ratio than men who have a higher muscle ratio. Fat retains heat better, thus men cool down faster than women. Men also feel more comfortable in cool air than women, due to differences in metabolism. Men's bodies release heat and women conserve heat.

The hands and feet of women are cooler than men, up to 3 degrees Fahrenheit cooler. The blood vessels in women's hands and feet constrict more than in men, thus making their hands and feet much colder.

The internal temperature in women fluctuates because of hormones, pregnancy, pills, etc.

In fact, a study in the science journal *Nature* done on Dutch women showed that 'on average, women in offices work better at a temperature 2.5°C warmer than men, generally falling somewhere between 24–25°C (75–77°F).'[1]

I met a couple where the woman keeps a heater on near her side of the bed while the husband has air conditioning on at room temperature 19 degrees Celsius.

Colour Preferences of Sheets

It is hard to believe but most women and men have a different colour preference of sheets—I once spoke to a lady who told me she preferred pink bedsheets while her husband wanted white!

Mattresses

Coming to the mattress . . . one wants it very firm and the other wants it very soft.

The resultant sleep disorders are, of course, very different.

Snoring

The habit of snoring in either partner interferes with the sleep of the other, causing insomnia. The entire night is spent agonizing, as the non-snoring partner is awake and is waiting for dawn. This results in arguments the next morning, each blaming the other. If this persists, then there is no choice but for one of the partners to shift to a separate bedroom, and in western countries it's even a reason for divorce.

Kicking

Kicking one's legs in sleep can disturb the other partner's sleep, as the kicking is usually repetitive in nature and very troublesome.

Shouting/Violent Behaviour in Sleep

This is known to occur in certain neuro-degenerative conditions. Such behaviour is extremely disturbing, with one partner suddenly experiencing a violent slap, or even being punched, by the other partner, or waking up to a blood-curdling loud scream.

How to Tackle This?

Change sleep timings, make arrangements for room temperature (different on either side), and change sleeping positions (one's head and the other's feet on either side of the bed) to avoid disturbing each other.

Does it Succeed? Not Really

There should be some better, permanent solution to the above problems. It is therefore best to consult a sleep specialist and seek solutions to maintain harmony in the bedroom and home.

For partners to continue to be in the same room and same bed, adjustments have to be made by each partner. Efforts to find a middle path for sleep timings and wake up timings, and adjusting the room temperature so that both partners feel comfortable are easy things to do.

For those who snore, kick, and shout in their sleep, it is important to meet a sleep specialist as these may be signs of a more sinister problem and should be treated not only to maintain relationships but also for ensuring good health.

Impact of Sleep Problems

We assess the impact in terms of direct and indirect costs.

Indirect Costs

- Interpersonal relations—with spouse, children, parents, colleagues—are greatly affected due to mood swings and irritability.

- Decreased interest in socializing.
- Frequent headaches.
- Frequent infections.

Direct Costs

> **Patients also reported that they felt sleepy while:**
> - Sitting idle
> - Watching TV
> - Talking to someone
> - Holding a phone (it suddenly slips from the hand)
> - Teaching
> - During a meeting
> - While counting money
> - Waiting for a flight at the airport (resulting in missing the flight or getting pick-pocketed)
> - While driving (resulting in having to pull over, take a nap or smoke)
> - In the washroom, especially at night (resulting in the door having to be broken down to get the patient out)
> - And believe it not, while making love!

- Frequent visits to the doctor due to additional complications such as high blood pressure, early onset of diabetes, heart and brain attacks, etc., which will require treatment and investigation.
- A patient revealed that he lost his job due to impaired productivity.
- Due to the increased sound of snoring, which disturbs fellow passengers, patients can't travel by bus or train; they have to travel solo by car.

- Sharing a room with such colleagues on business trips is a big issue. No one wants to share a room with them, so they end up taking a separate room and have to pay from their pockets!

Key Points for Better Sleep

- Sleep does affect relationships.
- Relationships can be affected by different preferences of partners, or two or more persons sharing the same room.
- Relationships can also be affected by real sleep disorders such as snoring, etc.
- The sleep time behaviour of partners can be extremely disturbing.
- It is therefore best to see a sleep specialist and seek solutions.

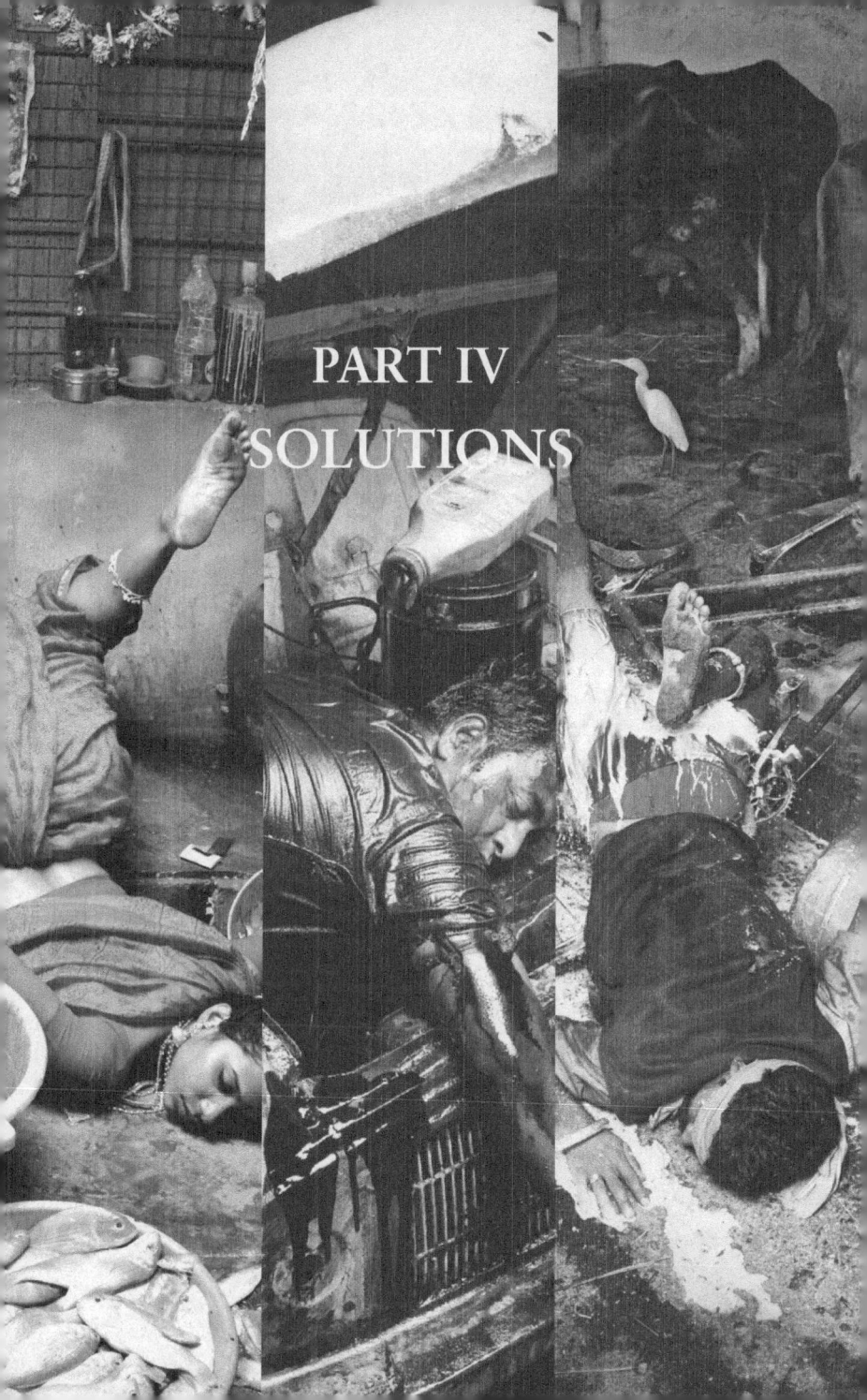

PART IV

SOLUTIONS

15

HOW CAN I SLEEP BETTER?

Are you interfering with your homeostatic drive by spending, for instance, a lot of time in bed during the day, especially taking long naps in the late afternoon? This will decrease your desire to sleep or your 'sleep drive'. But, before you panic and rush to a doctor, or start taking sleeping pills, as a sleep specialist, I would suggest you do two things. One, try to understand and learn what controls your sleep and wakefulness. Two, once you know a bit more about what controls your sleep and wakefulness, figure out what you're doing wrong to disrupt your own sleep.

WHAT DETERMINES SLEEPINESS?

There are two drives for inducing sleep: the homeostatic drive and the circadian drive.

Homeostatic Drive

The homeostatic drive is determined by how much one has slept the previous night. After a good night's rest, when we wake up in the morning, the desire to sleep and the sleep drive are low. In contrast, following a bad night, the desire to sleep and the sleep drive are high; overall, the tendency to fall asleep is strong.

Circadian Rhythm

The circadian rhythm is controlled by the pineal gland, the pacemaker which controls sleep and a host of other functions. It is low in the morning and increases towards the evening, with an increase in the drive in the afternoon as well. This explains the afternoon 'dip' and the desire for a nap. A variety of factors influence this, such as light and other somnogens (sleep-inducing substances)— adenosine, cytokines, etc. Anything which blocks the somnogens will interfere with sleep.

The Role of Melatonin

Melatonin is a hormone secreted by the pineal gland. It is responsible for controlling our sleep and waking up cycles, i.e. the internal clock of our body. Light and darkness are responsible for regulating the levels of melatonin in our body—light decreases and darkness increases these levels. This tells us why we fall asleep during night time. Melatonin levels drop with age. It also affects the female reproductive hormones. It determines the onset of the menstrual cycle, the duration of the cycle, etc., and also the age for menopause. By understanding what causes an increase and decrease in melatonin, we can understand the principles of sleep hygiene.

What Increases the Secretion of Melatonin?

An increase in the level of melatonin is inversely proportional to light. Therefore, darkening the environment before sleeping will help elevate the level of melatonin. To sleep better:

- One should always sleep in darkness.
- Excessive use of stimulants, like gadgets, should be avoided as it will lead to the suppression of melatonin.
- Foods like bananas, ginger, garlic, tomatoes, radishes and red wine should be consumed as they are natural sources of melatonin.
- Foods that contain tryptophan can also be eaten in the evening, as these help induce the production of serotonin, which is required to make melatonin. Dairy products, soy, seafood and nuts etc. are high in tryptophan.

What Decreases the Secretion of Melatonin?

The blue light emitted from laptops and cell phones interferes with the release of melatonin, thus causing insomnia. Gadgets should be switched off at least an hour prior to sleep, and should be kept at a distance while sleeping.

What Makes Us Wakeful?

One of the most important, yet often unasked, questions is what makes us wakeful and alert, and what makes us sleepy? The areas active in our brain are responsible for the different stages a person goes through during sleep.

The process is a complex one, as different parts of the brain simultaneously coordinate with each other and with an entire host of chemicals called neurotransmitters to ensure that the brain goes through these stages.

Neurotransmitters

Neurotransmitters (NT) are chemicals produced by nerve cells (neurons) in the brain. These NTs act on different groups of neurons to control the state of our mind when we are awake, as opposed to when we are asleep. In general, the areas in the brain responsible for producing wakefulness send signals to the cerebral cortex (the outer part of the brain, which controls thinking, learning, movement, etc.) and at the same time inhibits (decreases) activity in areas that promote sleep. A whole concoction of neurotransmitters is involved in driving wakefulness and sleep. The common ones are histamine, dopamine, norepinephrine, serotonin, glutamate, orexin and acetylcholine, among others.

Histamine

This is also known as the 'master' wakefulness-promoting neurotransmitter. It is increased when a person is awake and decreased during sleep. This makes it simple to understand how antihistamines cause sleepiness.

Serotonin

Serotonin activity promotes wakefulness, increases sleep onset latency (the length of time it takes to fall asleep) and decreases REM sleep.

Acetylcholine

Acetylcholine activity in the reticular activating system of the brainstem stimulates activity in the forebrain and cerebral cortex, encouraging alertness and wakefulness, although it also appears to be active during REM sleep.

Dopamine

The role of dopamine is very complex—depending on the receptors it acts on, it can cause wakefulness and sometimes even sleep.

Orexin

This is a recent discovery, but it plays an important role in the sleep–wake cycle. In fact, it affects many other functions, such as appetite, arousal, etc. This is produced by neurons in the hypothalamus and spread to many areas of the brain. Increased orexin causes wakefulness and a fall in its levels causes sleepiness and poor quality of sleep. Deficiency of orexin is the cause of a condition called narcolepsy. In fact, any tumour, head injury or stroke, which affects the orexin-producing neurons will result in sleepiness.

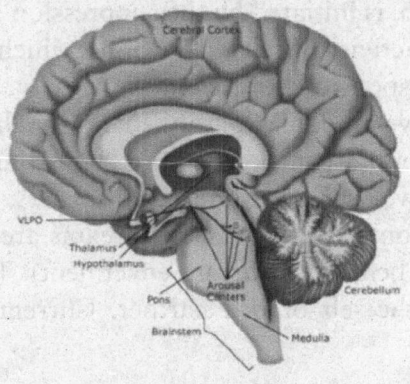

The arousal centres in the lower part of the brain keep us awake and inhibit the ventrolateralpreoptic nucleus (VLPO), which induces NREM sleep. VLPO, on the other hand, inhibits the wake-promoting centres and induces sleep.

Wakefulness is regulated by groups of neurons in the brain stem, hypothalamus and basal forebrain. They activate the thalamus (also called the gatekeeper), which sends impulses to the cortex, resulting in alerting a response. Thus, injury to this area or any medication which interferes with this function will cause increased sleepiness (anti-histamines for colds, etc. cause drowsiness).

The pre-optic area—VLPO—of the hypothalamus acts like a switch between sleep and wakefulness. When active, it induces sleep, inhibits wakefulness and initiates NREM sleep. The neurotransmitters are inhibitory. They inhibit the wake-promoting areas, decrease thalamo-cortical activation, causing initiation of sleep. Lesions in this area can cause insomnia or poor sleep.

It is now thought that there is a flip-flop switch via which the wakefulness- and sleep-promoting areas inhibit and activate each other. REM sleep, also called active sleep, is initiated by the suppression of orexin, and increased activity of cells in the pons, which also suppress the cells responsible for the motor activity. The result is a highly active brain in a 'paralysed' body. Though we have an increase in dreams during this stage, the body doesn't move. However, in certain sleep disorders, where there is degeneration of these cells, the dreams are accompanied by violent behaviour (dream enactment). This can cause injury to the self or bed partner. Current research has clearly shown that this condition can precede neuro-degenerative conditions, such as memory loss, imbalance and walking difficulties, by a decade.

How Does Coffee Affect Sleep?

The caffeine in coffee blocks adenosine receptors. To start with, we need to understand the function of adenosine. Adenosine levels increase during the day and on binding to receptors (a receptor a protein molecule that receives chemical signals from outside a cell), produce sleepiness. Caffeine mimics adenosine and, on binding to the receptor, produces a reverse reaction and instead of causing drowsiness, it causes wakefulness. The receptors can no longer identify adenosine because caffeine takes up all the receptors that adenosine would normally bind to.

As a result of this increased neuron firing, the pituitary gland releases more alerting hormones, adrenaline, that further causes stimulation.

Caffeine also affects dopamine production that makes us feel good. All these combine together to keep us awake and alert, preventing sleep.

Key Points for Better Sleep

- Darkening the environment before sleeping will help in elevating the level of melatonin—a hormone responsible for controlling our sleep and waking up cycles. One should always sleep in darkness.
- The blue light emitted from laptops and cell phones interferes with the release of melatonin, thus causing insomnia. Gadgets should be switched off at least

an hour prior to sleep, and kept at a distance while sleeping.

- Foods like bananas, ginger, garlic, tomatoes, radishes and red wine should be consumed as they are natural sources of melatonin.
- With all the stimulation that the caffeine in coffee provides, falling asleep is not easy. Therefore, generally, coffee is best avoided four–five hours before bedtime.
- Try and figure out what you're doing wrong to disrupt your own sleep.

16

SLEEP HYGIENE

What is sleep hygiene? It means those habits and behaviour that help us sleep well at night. It also comprises habits which impair sleep and need to be avoided.

As part of sleep hygiene, you should look out for three major factors:

- Body clock
- Relaxation and sleep
- Drugs and disruptive environment

Body Clock

This is a term for the biological clock inside our body, which controls various functions like sleep, wakefulness, appetite, hormone production, alertness, mood, etc.

This is an approximate twenty-four-hour clock/ cycle, also called the circadian rhythm, and exists in all species. Even when we're not at work, we're on the clock—our biological clock, that is. The strongest sleep drive for adults is between 2–4 a.m., and in the afternoon between 1–3 p.m. At other times of the day, the sleep drive is less, hence we feel more alert. The amount we sleep the preceding night also influences our sleep drive. Some body clock basics:

- Maintain regular hours for sleeping and waking up.
- Avoid variations of over two hours in the waking up time on weekends.
- Avoid staying in bed for over 7.5 hours.
- Exercise daily, but at least 4–5 hours before sleeping.

Relaxation and Sleep

Relaxation and sleep are an important part of sleep hygiene. As a sleep specialist, I advise you to:

- Avoid emotionally disturbing activities near bedtime (disturbing pillow talk).
- Avoid any kind of activity that demands high concentration immediately before going to bed.
- Avoid mental activities such as thinking, planning or recollecting in bed.

Drugs and Disruptive Environment

We don't realize it but drugs and disruptive environments make us irritable in life. We make them a part of our lives and they take life away from us. There are a few myths about these things, which should be taken care of for a healthy life.

Prior to sleeping, avoid products that contain:

- **Alcohol:** It's a common belief that alcohol induces sleep. Yes, this is partly true. As it is a depressant, it slows down the nervous system. It does help in the onset of sleep, but it does disturb the sleep quality, causing breaks in sleep (fragmentation). This leads to us waking up feeling tired and not particularly refreshed in the morning. Excessive alcohol intake can also cause frequent trips to the washroom and a hangover the next day.
- **Tobacco:** It is often thought that smoking is relaxing, but nicotine has a stimulant effect. It causes an increase in the heart rate and blood pressure, causing a delay in the onset of sleep.
- **Sleeping pills:** As the name suggests, sleeping pills help one fall asleep faster. Some of these have a very long duration of action and cause daytime sleepiness or a hangover-like effect. After using pills for some time, it is difficult to fall asleep without pills. Prolonged use is harmful as the dosage has to be increased to produce the desired effect. They should be used only for a short time and under the supervision of a specialist. Never self-medicate.
- **Caffeine:** This blocks the actions of sleep-inducing substances, causing wakefulness.

Things to Remember

- 'Sleep hygiene' means habits that help you have a good night's sleep.

- Common sleeping problems (such as insomnia) are often caused by bad habits reinforced over the years or even decades.
- If you have tried and failed to improve your sleep, you may like to consider professional help.

Some do's and don'ts which improve the quality of sleep.

Do's
- Get a new pillow.
- Do open blinds and curtains when you wake up.
- Only go to bed when you are feeling sleepy.
- Get some exercise during the day.
- Spend some time outdoors, in sunlight or natural light.
- Make the bedroom as restful as possible.
- Develop a routine before bed (brushing your teeth, drinking warm milk, light reading, relaxation or breathing exercises).
- Get yourself organized for the next day—pack your bag, get your clothes ready, organize your lunch, etc.
- Use your bedroom for sleep only!

Don'ts
- Don't watch TV or play on your computer too close to bedtime.
- Don't eat protein too late at night.
- Don't consume stimulants in the afternoon—no coffee, tea, cola, energy drinks, chocolate, nicotine, alcohol, etc., after 3.p.m.
- Don't stay in bed if you're awake; if you're still awake twenty–thirty minutes after going to bed, get up and

do something boring in dim light until you feel sleepy again.

- Don't keep looking at the clock. This can make things worse and make you feel even more frustrated that you're not asleep yet! If you need your clock for an alarm, turn it around, so you aren't tempted to look at it. Even better, remove it from your room completely!

Your Pre-bedtime Routine

You may be one of the many who are unable to fall asleep quickly. If you choose to neglect this problem, your body and mind are more likely to suffer. Recent research has shown that people with symptoms of insomnia, also suffer from mental issues like depression and anxiety. Other diseases one may suffer from include diabetes and congestive heart failure.

However, there is no reason to panic. Sleep routines can be easily fixed through regularly practiced relaxation techniques, like yoga and chanting.

If you are a beginner, it is advisable to do each of the following yoga poses at least five times, in order to familiarize yourself with them. If some of these poses are uncomfortable for you, try picking your favourite five and repeat them every day in order to establish a routine. These poses can be practiced even in bed. Always keep in mind that these exercises are meant for relaxation; pushing yourself outside your comfort zone could be harmful. Contact a yoga practitioner before modifying or experimenting with any of the following poses.

Janu Sirsasana (Head-to-knee Pose)

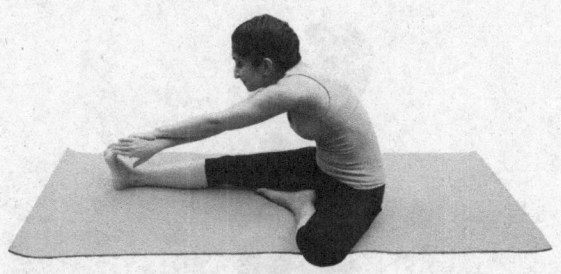

- Sit with a straight back and stretch your legs in front of you, making sure that your spine is comfortable. For the convenience of your spine, bending your knees is a viable option.
- Gently angle your right leg in such a way that your right foot touches the muscles of your inner left thigh. For the sake of convenience, you can use a small pillow or a padded cushion to support your right knee properly.
- Monitor your breathing. Stretch your spine as you inhale and then exhale. Stretch out to your left foot with both hands, making sure that your focus on your left foot does not hamper your straight neck and back, now at an acute angle. Hold this position and resume your breathing.
- Now gently let go of this position. Outstretch your right leg again and repeat this exercise on the left side.

Make it easier: Use a small pillow or cushion to support your knees

Baddha Konasana (Bound Angle Pose)

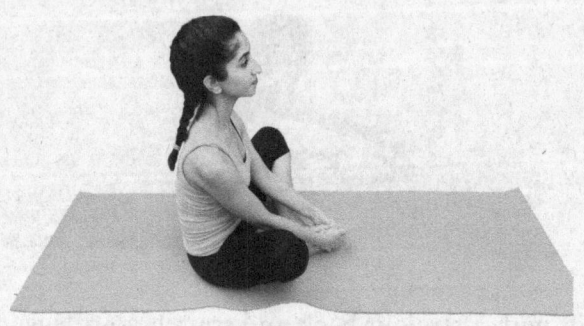

- Sit straight in a cross-legged position and then, gently bring the soles of your feet together while you hold your ankles in order to maintain this position.
- If convenient, bring your joined feet as close to your pelvic region as possible, without risking any pressure on your back.
- If your spine slouches, inhale deeply and straighten your back.
- While keeping your spine straight, exhale deeply while angling yourself forward. Hold this position and continue to breathe normally.

Make it easier: Use a small pillow or a padded cushion and place it under your hips in order to help you bend. If your spine is still strained, avoid bending.

Upavistha Konasana (Wide-angle Seated Forward Bend)

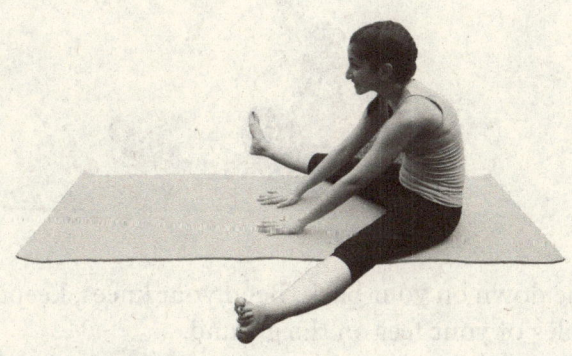

- Sit still, keeping back straight.
- Stretch your legs out in front of you. Gently swing your legs outwards to form a 'V', making sure your hamstrings are not strained.
- Make sure your spine is not bent. If it is, take a deep breath and straighten your back.
- Place your hands inside this 'V' position and bend forward while exhaling deeply. Monitor your breathing. Straighten your back with an inhalation and loosen the pressure as you bend forward and exhale.

Make it easier: Use your hands or a small pillow in order to support your buttocks, especially while bending forwards. However, if you continue to feel excessive strain on your hamstrings, it is advisable to avoid bending altogether.

Thread-the-needle

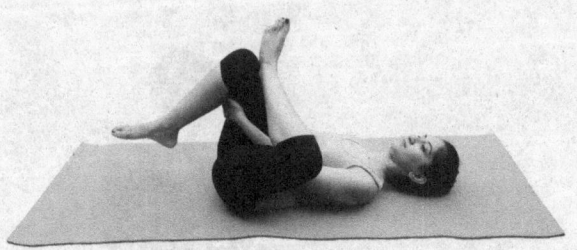

- Lie down on your back. Bend your knees, keeping the soles of your feet on the ground.
- Without straining yourself, bend your right leg and then place your right ankle below your left knee. The right foot must not be held in a stagnant position. Flex your right foot to ensure pressure does not build on your right knee.
- Now lift off your left sole from the ground so that your left knee is angled towards your chest. For ease, place both of your hands on the floor as your right hip continues to be stretched. Take deep breaths and try to keep your hips even.

Ease back to the first step, and then, repeat the exercise on the other side.

Reclined Twist

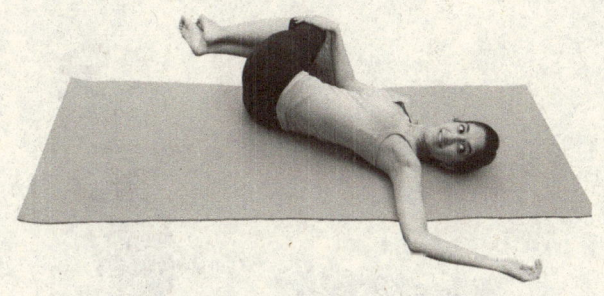

- Lie down on your back. Now, angle your knees in such a position that they are touching your chest.
- Stretch your left arm towards your shoulder, palm up.
- Hold the position and then gently swing your knees towards your right until they touch the floor.
- In order to hold your position, use your right hand and place it on the top of the right knee. You can also massage your outer leg to ease the pressure.
- Keep your gaze focused on the ceiling above or towards your left.
- Ease back and then repeat this exercise on the other side.

Make it easier: While your knees are touching the ground, put a small pillow or a padded cushion under your legs so that the strain is eased.

Viparita Karani (Legs-against-the-wall Pose)

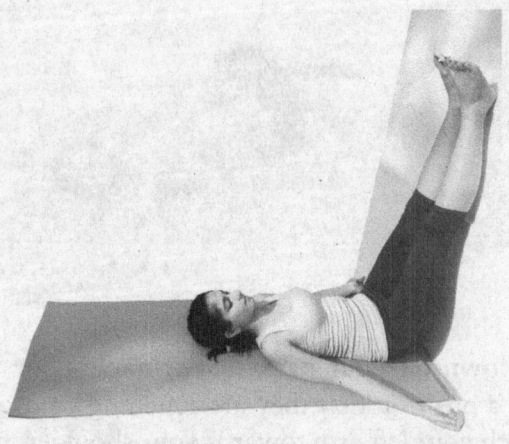

- Lie down on the floor, with your feet facing the wall. Raise one leg horizontally, so that it touches the wall. Next, raise the other leg so that both your legs are in a 90 degree position against the wall.
- Stretch your arms out on each side, palms up.
- Relax and close your eyes. For convenience, use an eye-pillow so that bright lights do not hinder your relaxation.

Make it easier: Instead of a complete 90 degree angle, move your hips away from the wall so that the pressure on your hamstrings is eased. You can also tie your lower legs to make the pose more comfortable.

Winding Down Twist

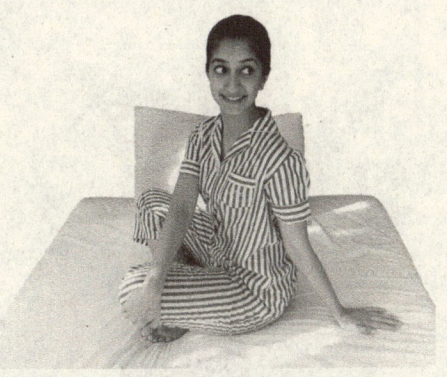

- Sit in a relaxed cross-legged position, while monitoring your breathing. Place your right hand on your left knee and exhale deeply. Place your other hand behind your hips.
- Swinging towards your left hand, gently shift your torso towards your left.
- Shift your gaze towards your left shoulder and take a deep breath. Now, gently move back to the centre. Repeat the exercise on the other side.

Night-time Goddess Stretch

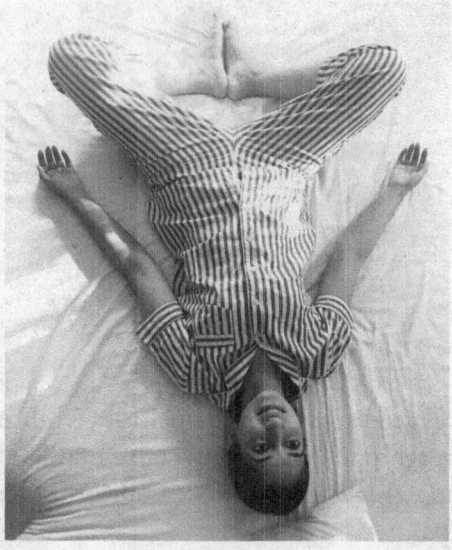

- Lie down with your back on the bed. Make sure that your knees are bent.
- Open your knees out and bring the soles of your feet together, so that they touch. Your lower body should form a diamond position of sorts.
- Relax your arms on each side.
- For convenience, place a small pillow or a padded cushion underneath your knees.

Child Pose

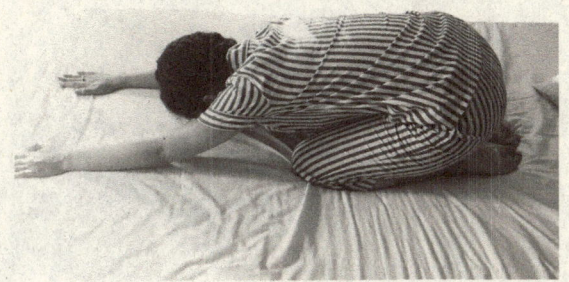

- Sit on your heels, making sure that you are comfortable.
- Gently bend forward with the help of your torso, so that your forehead touches the bed.
- Extend your arms in front of your forehead and at the same time, lower your chest so that it touches your knees.
- Relax, hold the position and breathe.

Rock-a-bye Roll

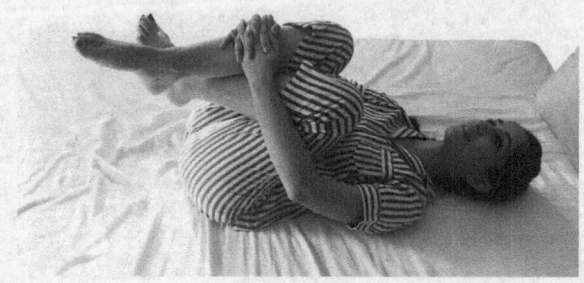

- Lie down on your back and bring your knees up to your chest.
- Gently, cross your ankles and wrap your hands around your shins to hold your legs in place.
- Monitor your breathing. Inhale as you roll on to the sitting-up position and exhale as you roll back to your back.
- Carry on like this for about a minute, exhale, roll back and then gently extend your limbs in order to sleep.

Chanting

Chanting is an excellent method to relax before sleep. Usually associated with religious rituals, it is a way to ensure peace in the lives of people who are looking for contentment—religious or not. While mysticism might draw some people towards chanting, some people may not be comfortable with it.

Chanting does not only offer mental relaxation, it is also known to help the physical transformation of bodies via which the internal systems are recharged and made healthy again. It lowers blood pressure, channels brain waves into calmness, and also helps produce melatonin, which is an excellent agent for sleep. Therefore, it can definitely help improve our sleeping patterns.

Further, research shows that chanting is beneficial for both halves of the brain. The left half is usually the dominant part, associated with analysis, logical processing as well as facts and data. The right half, on the other hand, is associated with imagination and creative potential. Chanting helps unify both halves, thereby providing a complete sense of equilibrium.

A beginner's class will prove helpful, if you want to take up chanting. Online resources such as video tutorials can also be beneficial.

Apart from chanting, shavasana and pranayama are also excellent pre-sleep rituals. Shavasana allows you to let go the tension or nervousness building up in the muscles, which often cause pain and spasms. It is like resetting your body. It is very easy to practice and has many benefits.

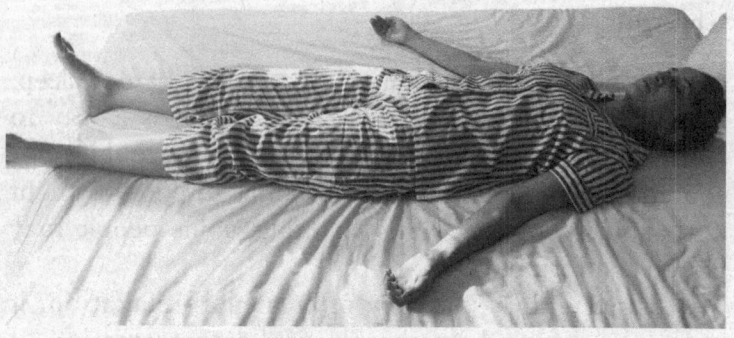

Make sure you are in a quiet place. Lie down on a mat on the floor. Loosen any tight clothing. Make sure the place is quiet, and switch off your phone and tablet. The lights should be either off or very dim. The room should be airy, so that you do not feel any difficulty in breathing.

Loosen your muscles. Relax your mind and body. The mind is similar to an overhead tank. Mentally, feel every part of your body. Begin with your feet.

Another way to relax the mind and body is through pranayama asana. 'Prana' refers to the vital energy that sustains the body in terms of function and activity. In other words, prana is what keeps our body alive. Pranayama is a way of controlling of that energy.

Here are some benefits of pranayama, which help in maintaining a balanced quality of life:

Pranayama Practice Increases Life

A certain yoga philosophy preaches that lowering your breathing rate may improve your life expectancy Tortoises, for instance, take only four to five breaths in one minute and live for a hundred years or more.

Improves Blood Circulation

Balanced breathing helps oxygenate your blood, which travels from the lungs to the heart resulting in with improved circulation. The heart pumps this blood and releases it in the blood vessels, which cover our entire body. Better blood circulation means higher levels of prana or cosmic energy.

Pranayama for a Healthy Heart

The heart is an indispensable organ as it manages the laborious function of keeping us alive. A healthy heart beats 1,00,000 times a day, without pausing for a single moment. It ensures longevity in terms of life expectancy as well as quality of life. More oxygen means more strength to the heart muscles.

Benefits of Pranayama for Functioning of Body Organs

Pranayama also helps a person deal with mental problems like anger, depression, lust, greed, arrogance, etc.

The mind can be put at ease and chaos can be dispelled through pranayama. With regular practice, the body experiences deep-rooted peace, better memory, good focus, as well as good sleep. It is also connected to improving an individual's spirituality.

Better Breathing Improves Quality of Life in Old Age

Lung problems can also be cured through pranayama. As an effect of old age, weakness in the lungs often causes problems in an otherwise healthy life. Pranayama ensures that lungs function properly, despite modern lifestyles.

A yoga teacher will be able to help you master the practice of pranayama. With experience, the technique will become smoother and more beneficial. A daily routine of such breathing exercises is highly advisable. Concentrate on your breathing rhythms, and make it deeper with every inhalation and exhalation.

EPILOGUE

Sleep is a subject that can't be wished away. No matter what one's age is, sleep is essential for all. Getting good sleep and getting enough sleep are interlinked and vital for us to function optimally. The good thing is, there is enough information and a remedy for all kinds of sleep disorders. Understanding the 'why' and 'how' of sleep is most important. This book is an attempt to provide you with comprehensive information on all aspects of sleep.

Sleep needs and daily requirement differs from person to person. A few people need less sleep and some need more—figure out how much you need and strive towards achieving it.

I had a lady visit me once. She was forty-two years old, and worked from 8 a.m. to 10 p.m. She would get only five–six hours of sleep at night, and started developing palpitations, constrictions in the chest and intermittent difficulty in breathing at night. All the tests she underwent said she was normal. She then came to me normal. On being questioned, she said she was initially very keen on her job, but had become unhappy as it ate away the little personal time she had for herself.

We all find ourselves slowly prolonging our day, push without realizing our limits. But what we don't realize is that this impacts the quality and quantity of our sleep, resulting in anxiety, mood changes and, ultimately, it leads to low productivity.

I hope I've convinced you about the magic of sleep through this book. If you picked up this book, it means that you want to understand sleep or solve sleep issues. Hopefully, the purpose was achieved. The stories of my patients continue to surprise me and solving their problems often fills me with emotions hard to describe. I've attempted to cover many common and uncommon issues related to sleep, so that you can relate to the different issues and the solutions offered in the book.

My vision for the future is that we, as a community—adults, children, employers, truckers, pilots, entrepreneurs—understand the importance of sleep. Even companies like Google have mandated sleep hours for their employees. Something as simple as good sleep can prevent many illnesses—mental and physical—and promote overall health and make people happier. I am already working on other books on sleep benefits, like beauty through sleep, good sleep through correct diet, sleep and a better lifestyle, sleep for different ages and genders, and so on. I sincerely hope that through this book I have been able to provide answers to all your sleep problems.

Here's wishing you a good night's sleep!

AFTERWORD

It gives me great pleasure to write the afterword for *The Sleep Solution*, a comprehensive and concise book, written by my esteemed colleague, Dr Manvir Bhatia, whom I have known for almost twenty years. In this easy-to-read book, she has tackled the seemingly simple, but rather complex, state of human existence—sleep, that mysterious state of being and that gentle tyrant—in a lucid manner.

The book offers a wealth of wisdom—distilled from her extensive experience in dealing with patients who share the common complaints of 'Doctor, I can't sleep', 'I sleep too much', 'I can't sleep at the right time', 'I have weird dreams or move excessively during sleep'. In this book, she has gone through these problems and their solutions step by step—from making a correct diagnosis to the final step of finding a solution—in a very simple way for the layperson and for those interested in the subject.

Written in a thoughtful and practical manner that distils the complex issues of sleep dysfunction, this book will serve as an invaluable source for those who are afflicted by sleep disorders (individuals personally or family members, friends and co-workers). The book will also be useful to physicians, who are just beginning to understand the mystery of sleep and how to approach a very common problem (often a challenge to treat) in the field of sleep medicine.

I would like to end by recounting what Raman Maharshi said when one of his disciples asked, 'What is sleep?' Maharshi said, 'You must ask this question in sleep.' Confused, the disciple asked, 'How can I do that in sleep?' But Maharshi insisted that the question should be raised only in sleep. The disciple pressed on, 'I cannot ask that question in sleep.' To that, Maharshi said, 'Well, that is what sleep is.'

Despite years of intense research, we still cannot answer the pertinent questions of 'What is sleep?' 'Why do we sleep?' 'How do we remain awake?' At the end of this concise compendium, I guarantee that you will be enlightened about sleep, its disorders, how to approach the problem and how to tackle the very common problem of sleep difficulty in our modern society by using some simple alternative measures suggested rather than depending on medications with their inherent adverse effects.

A great deal of wisdom has been compressed in this book, as illustrated by the numerous clinical vignettes derived from cases in the real world, tackled over the years by Dr Bhatia in a most masterful manner.

Sudhansu Chokroverty, MD, FRCP, FACP
Seton Hall University, South Orange, New Jersey
JFK New Jersey Neuroscience Institute, Edison, New Jersey
Rutgers Robert Wood Johnson Medical School, New Brunswick, New Jersey

REFERENCES

Chapter 1
What is Sleep?

1. 'Insufficient Sleep Is a Public Health Problem', http://www.cdc.gov/features/dssleep/

Chapter 2
Why Do We Sleep?

1. 'Take that Nap', http://sharpbrains.com/blog/2010/10/18/take-that-nap-it-may-boost-your-learningcapacity-among-other-good-things/

Chapter 5
Effects of Sleep Deprivation and Sleep Debt

1. 'How Much Sleep do We Need?' http://www.howsleepworks.com/need_debt.html

2. 'Short sleep duration, sleep disorders, and traffic accidents', http://www.sciencedirect.com/science/article/pii/S0386111213000149

3. 'Driver's Working Time', http://tachospeed.com/legal/regulation-no-5612006-drivers-working-time-2/

4. 'New Pilot Fatigue Rules go into Effect This Weekend', http://www.usatoday.com/story/todayinthesky/2014/01/03/pilot-fatigue-mandatory-rest-new-faa-rules/4304417/

5. 'Do History's Greatest Figures owe their Success to Sleeping Less?', http://www.nydailynews.com/historygreatest-figures-owe-success-sleeping-article-1.412799

Chapter 6
Can Sleep Be Measured?

1. Chung F., Yegneswaran B., Liao P., Chung S.A., Vairavanathan S., Islam S., et al. STOP questionnaire: a tool to screen patients for obstructive sleep apnea. Anesthesiology. 2008 May; 108(5):812–21.

2. Murray W. Johns. 'A New Method For Measuring Daytime Sleepiness: The Epworth Sleepiness Scale'. *Sleep*. 1991;14(06):540–5.

3. Netzer N.C., Stoohs R.A., Netzer C.M., Clark K., Strohl K.P. Using the Berlin Questionnaire to identify patients at risk for the sleep apnea syndrome. Ann Intern Med. 1999 Oct 5; 131(7):485–91.

4. Buysse D.J., Reynolds C.F., Monk T.H., Berman S.R., Kupfer D.J. The Pittsburgh Sleep Quality Index: a new instrument for psychiatric practice and research. Psychiatry Res. 1989 May; 28(2):193–213.

Chapter 7
Sleep and Health

1. 'The Impact of Sleep Deprivation on Hormones and Metabolism', http://www.medscape.org/viewarticle/502825
2. 'The Link between Short Sleep Duration and Obesity', http://www.ncbi.nlm.nih.gov/pmc/articles/PMC2082964/

Chapter 8
Sleep and Beauty

1. 'How Naps can Improve your Skin', http://www.howtogetrid.org/beauty/how-naps-can-improve-yourskin/
2. 'Sleeping Beauty: Sleep Your Way to Better Skin and Hair', http://www.fitnessmagazine.com/beauty/hair/sleeping-beauty-sleep-your-way-to-better-skin-andhair/
3. 'Beautiful Skin Begins with a Good Night's Sleep', http://www.nyrnaturalnews.com/article/getting-yourbeauty-sleep/
4. '6 Amazing Reasons to Sleep for Skin Health', http://www.huffingtonpost.com/entry/skin-caresleep_n_2806573.html?section=india&utm_hp_ref=tw
5. 'Beauty Sleep is Real', http://www.alaskasleep.com/blog/beauty-sleep-is-real.-how-lack-of-sleep-is-ruining-your-skin
6. 'Are You Getting Enough Beauty Sleep?', https://bhi.edu/getting-enough-beauty-sleep/

Chapter 9
Sleep and Food

1. 'Studies on Health', https://ibstreatmentcenter.com/tag/studies-on-health
2. 'Sleep Influences Food Intake', https://healthesolutions.com/sleep-influences-food-intake/

Chapter 10
Common Sleep Disorders

1. 'Sleep Disorders and Sleep Deprivation', http://www.ncbi.nlm.nih.gov/books/NBK19961/

Chapter 11
Sleep and Technology

1. 'Will a Gadget Help you Sleep?', http://www.webmd.com/women/features/sleep-gadgets-apps-tips?page=1

Chapter 14
Sleep and Relationships

1. 'Do Women Get Colder than Men?' http://www.bustle.com/articles/102194-do-women-get-colder-than-menwhy-freezing-offices-are-worse-for-us

ACKNOWLEDGEMENTS

There are a few things one grows up thinking one should do some day, and writing a book was one of those for me.

For years, I was fascinated by the various stories related to sleep issues that I heard from patients every day at my clinic. I started keeping a journal, sometimes even recording their voices, hoping that someday I would be able to write about them in a book. Despite the fact the Internet has a lot of information about sleep, a large number of patients felt it was not enough and wanted more authentic information. This prompted me to write a book on the topic.

I mentioned this to my friends George and Sarah, who introduced me to Dilip Cherian. After that things moved very fast. Dilip introduced me to the good folks at Penguin Random House India, and everything fell into place thereafter.

I was filled with apprehension, as this is my first book. However, with continuous encouragement from my husband—who has always motivated me to chase my dreams—and from my family, friends and patients, I finally decided to give it a shot.

But writing a book is no easy task and I was ably guided along the way by a whole team.

Firstly, a big thank you to my patients, without whom I wouldn't even have had the idea of writing a book.

To my mother, who has always been there to help, encourage and guide me through every stage of my life. To Anubha, Nivedita and Veenu, for helping me with the research. Padma, who took the time to go through the draft numerous times, and my colleagues at ISB, for their suggestions and support. Special thanks to Divya, who pushed me to complete the draft. To Gurveen, for her constant support and encouragement. And finally, to all my friends for their support and belief in me.

ABOUT THE AUTHOR

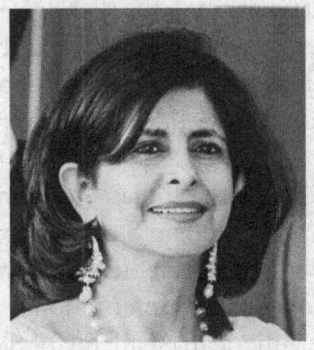

Dr Manvir Bhatia is India's leading sleep specialist and neurologist. She is the director of sleep medicine at the Neurology Sleep Centre, Delhi, and also at the Fortis Escorts Heart Institute, Delhi. She completed her post-graduation from the All India Institute of Medical Sciences (AIIMS), New Delhi, in the department of neurology, and her MBBS and MD (medicine) from CMCH, Ludhiana. She was also awarded a scholarship and prize for the '10,000 Women' certificate programme for women entrepreneurs by Goldman Sachs, at ISB, Hyderabad. She is also the recipient of the Indira Gandhi Mahila Ratan Award, 2016.

Dr Bhatia is a member of the executive committee of the Indian Sleep Disorders Association and the Indian Sleep Research Society. She was invited by the WHO to help develop guidelines on health issues related to sleep. She has initiated a training programme for doctors in sleep medicine and is a pioneer in creating awareness about sleep disorders and establishing the role of sleep medicine in the country.

Dr Bhatia has been invited to deliver lectures in both national and international workshops, conferences on topics related to neurology, epilepsy and sleep medicine. She has also published more than eighty papers in leading journals and has authored several chapters in various books.

She is a member of the Indian Academy of Neurology, Indian Epilepsy Society, Indian Sleep Disorders Association, World Association of Sleep Medicine, International Restless Legs Society Study Group, International Paediatric Sleep Academy and the American Academy of Sleep Medicine.

The Sleep Solution is her first book.

She can be reached at: neurologysleepcentre@gmail.com, info@neurologysleepcentre.com

Her website is: www.neurologysleepcentre.com; www.sleepapnoeaindia.com